the
DETOX
FACTOR

101 TIPS & TRICKS TO LOSE WEIGHT WITHOUT DIETING

(PRINT EDITION – ENGLISH, UK)

- ANGIE NEWSON -

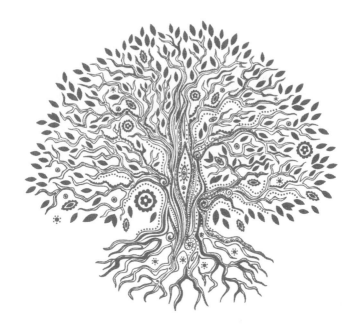

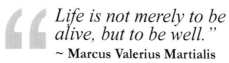

Life is not merely to be alive, but to be well. "
~ **Marcus Valerius Martialis**

I dedicate this book to everyone who chooses to beautify their body from the inside. To those who want to live an honest and authentic life — full of love, clarity and peace of mind.

We are souls at different stages on our paths, yet all playing the same game. Here's to a long, happy and healthy journey.

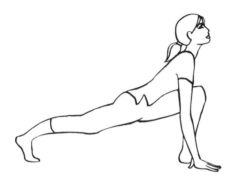

Live in rooms full of light

Avoid heavy food

Be moderate in the drinking of wine

*Take massage, baths,
exercise and gymnastics*

*Fight insomnia with gentle rocking
or the sound of running water*

*Change surroundings and
take long journeys*

Strictly avoid frightening ideas

*Indulge in cheerful conversation
and amusements*

Listen to music."
~ **Aulus Cornelius Celsus**

WHY I WROTE THIS BOOK

I f you want to finally shift that stubborn belly fat and banish frequent colds and flu then this book is for you. If you have difficulty sleeping, pounding headaches or digestive issues, then my tips will help you get on the right track to optimal healthy living – naturally. I've always been interested in clean eating, and throughout my long career in the wellbeing industry, apart from joyously advocating the valuable and obvious benefits of exercise, I also promote a wholesome and nourishing diet. I've brought up a family, taught over 11,000 fitness classes (and still counting), and the one big question I'm asked constantly is how to lose weight and keep it off for good. I reveal my secrets of effortless weight loss and what you can do to improve your vitality and confidence so you feel sexy and alive again.

I've been detoxing for many years now and continue to regularly cleanse, physically and mentally, profiting from the worthwhile perks. You too will find that by detoxing your body – and your mind – you become more grounded, you'll be an inspiration to your friends and have bags more energy. Retraining your taste buds and eating the right foods, in the right quantities and at the right speed, is vital to how you feel, how you look and how you function. My detoxifying, healthy way of living will naturally slim your waist, boost your immune system, soothe your digestion and enhance your longevity.

No doubt, some days may be easier than others – resist beating yourself up about it. As Oscar Wilde said *'What seems to us as bitter trials are often blessings in disguise.'* I guarantee that once you're in the full flow of clean living, receiving admiring compliments and looking more youthful – you'll be championing my secrets and some of your own too!

WHY READ THIS BOOK

This book offers easy-to-follow tips to motivate you to lead a cleaner lifestyle – changes you can make immediately – simple and yet powerful solutions to enhance your life and clear toxicity. It's a practical guide to improve your diet, looks and everyday wellbeing. These pointers work for me and my clients and I'm delighted to pass them on to you. Take what you want and leave the rest. I am very pro-choice – remember you are the boss of you – use your innate intuition to empower your life!

HERE ARE SOME OF THE HEALTH PERKS YOU WILL GAIN
You will ...

- *Get rid of that annoying belly fat.*

- *Look younger than your actual age.*

- *Have smooth digestion without any bloating or gas.*

- *Crave healthy food that empowers your wellbeing.*

- *Have boundless energy throughout the day.*

- *Be mentally alert without any 'brain fog'.*

- *Sleep soundly and feel energised on awakening.*

- *Be happy and content without any mood swings.*

PRAISE FOR *THE DETOX FACTOR*

'Great read! It manages to stay light; yet it is informative, well researched, insightful and full of little pearls to help us all live cleaner and longer lives'
Peter Gould / CEO Great Hotels of the World, London, UK

'This book gets straight to the point of changes that can be implemented immediately to detox and cleanse. An amazing source of information about anti-ageing and weight loss too.'
Teka Bury / Owner of Bikram Yoga, Ipanema, Rio de Janeiro, Brazil

'This detox and cleanse guide has helped me make simple changes to my diet to improve my lifestyle and energy levels. I loved this book.'
Giles Bury / 9-times awarded film editor, Los Angeles, USA

'What a gem! Not too technical and written in an 'easy for the layperson to follow' style, Angie's straightforward approach demystifies the topics and instead of appearing as a 'mountain to climb', each step looks like a small hill instead!'
Emma Heaney / Director, Lettings Agent, Hertfordshire, UK

'This book has helped me make immediate lifestyle changes so much so that I'm now feeling revitalised and extremely positive. I have even started yoga and Pilates.'
David Elliott, Director of Landhold Developments Ltd, London, UK

'At last I can sit and read one book that answers all my questions. I have books for this, books for that and books for, well, everything else! This is a book full of great tips and information, which is extremely easy to read.'
Pat De Felice, Legal PA, Hertfordshire, UK

 The greatest wealth is health."
~ **Virgil**

PUBLISHER'S NOTE

This publication is intended to provide helpful and informative material. It is not intended to diagnose, treat, cure or prevent any health problem or condition, nor is intended to replace the advice of a physician. No action should be taken solely on the contents of this book. Always consult your physician or qualified health-care professional on any matters regarding your health and before adopting any suggestions in this book or drawing inferences from it.

The author and publisher specifically disclaim all responsibility for any liability, loss or risk, personal or otherwise, which is incurred as a consequence, directly or indirectly, from the use or application of any of the contents of this book.

Any and all product names referenced within this book are the trademarks of their respective owners. None of these owners have sponsored, authorised, endorsed or approved this book.

Always read all information provided by the manufacturers' product labels before using their products. The author and publisher are not responsible for claims made by manufacturers.

CONTENTS

THREE: LOVE YOUR LIVER

FOUR: BREATH OF LIFE   91

HOW TO USE THIS BOOK – THE DAILY DETOX

You can either read from beginning to end or flick through to the chapter that seems most relevant to what you want to change – or take pot-luck and pick a random topic from the contents list each day to learn something new!

I've designed this book to be a practical guide to boosting your body's natural ability and desire to do what I call a *'Daily Detox'*. By using the tips inside to make little daily changes to your lifestyle, you'll soon be reaping big rewards and living a longer, healthier life.

Just a reminder though – our mind and our body are inter-connected – we need a clear mind to keep motivation high enough to follow through with our Daily Detox desires, as well as a cleansed and healthy body to fuel and keep our mind alert.

I am a firm believer in Dr Bernard Jenson's ominous quote *'Death begins in the colon!'* (only if you let it though!) – so I highly recommend making gut health your number one priority for overall wellbeing.

Here are my top seven Daily Detox habits that were, for me, 'aha moments' when I first learned about them. Simply blending these ridiculously straightforward and cleanse-smart ideas into your life will be totally game-changing for your wellness – they certainly were for me!

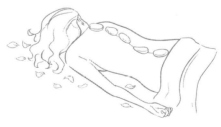

TOP SEVEN DAILY DETOX HABITS

#1 Banish	*Junk Food / Bad Pharma / Sugar*
#2 Nourish	*Organic Food / Good Fats / Fibre / Probiotics*
#3 Drink	*Water / Green Juices / Green Smoothies*
#4 Rest	*Sleep / Mindfulness / Meditation*
#5 Move	*HIIT / Rebounding / Dynamic Yoga*
#6 Nature	*Daylight / Breathe / Swimming*
#7 Wellbeing	*Massage / Cold Water Therapy / Infrared Sauna*

WHY CLEANSE?

Think of your body like your car – it needs regular maintenance, servicing, filter and oil changes, otherwise it doesn't run smoothly. Lack of care and attention means it will eventually break down and end up on the scrap heap. Similarly, we need to love our bodies – detoxing periodically and fuelling with nourishing and replenishing foods so we too can function and run smoothly. By combining this awareness with movement, yogic breathing and meditation, we can avoid our own scrap heap!

Removing toxins from our bodies helps prevent disease, boosts our immune system and aids tranquil digestion. Sleep is improved and you'll notice your complexion become clear and youthful. You'll have enhanced mental and emotional clarity, be able to focus and concentrate better and may even become more creative and artistic to boot!

Cleansing helps us live our lives at peak performance level – effortlessly – with renewed vigour, vibrancy and restored equilibrium. Aches and pains ease, unwanted pounds melt away and miraculously it becomes easy to maintain an ideal weight without ever needing a fad-diet again. Longevity here we come!

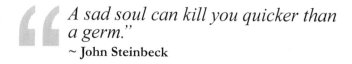 *A sad soul can kill you quicker than a germ."*
~ **John Steinbeck**

WHERE DO THE TOXINS COME FROM?

Our environment, the foods we eat, what we drink, legal and illegal drugs, stress, not enough exercise and an unhealthy lifestyle all go towards making our bodies toxic. We can also become emotionally and mentally toxic – full of negative thoughts, critical judgements of others and ourselves, and loaded down with heavy emotions such as anger or jealousy – causing our body's pH to slide to the acid end of the scale. We may also be living our lives surrounded by clutter and hoarding, along with a constant desire to continually get even more stuff that won't ever be used.

The air outside is full of carbon monoxide, pesticides, sulphur, lead and chemical fertilisers, to name just a few of the toxins we breathe in – particularly in cities and near airports. Inside our houses it's even more toxic as we inhale vapours from fire-retardant furniture, household chemical cleaners, dry-cleaned clothes, plastics, deodorants, air fresheners and even some scented candles and incense! The list is endless.

What we put on our skin also can be detrimental to our health – hair dyes, perfumes, make-up, creams, shampoos and even toothpaste can be harmful. It's not a case of scaremongering – it's about having the awareness and the know-how to minimise exposure to these impurities by reading the contents on labels, resist using aerosols, and buying organic creams and body products instead. Even better, delight in making your own beauty goodies at home so you really know what goes in them.

Learning how to reduce the negative effects of environmental pollutants that attack us from every angle every single day is vital – from being on our mobile phone too much or glued to our computer screens, to the chemical killers we put on the weeds in the garden – let's aim to seek natural ways to rectify this damage to ourselves and our world.

And what about our tap water? It may contain fluoride, chlorine and radioactive radon, and apart from absorbing water when we drink it, we shower in it, wash our hair in it and brush our teeth with it. Ideally having a water filter system fitted under your sink or at least using a water-filter jug for drinking water and teeth brushing will eliminate the impurities so our water is cleaner and safer to use.

Be mindful of the food you eat – buy organic fruit and veggies, or if this isn't always viable, ensure you wash your fresh produce well in a bowl of water containing a tablespoon of apple cider vinegar to get rid of the pesticides and chemical fertilisers. Better still – grow your own fruit and veggies!

The cheap cuts of meat, poultry and fish available in the stores today contain harmful amounts of growth hormones, antibiotics and steroids – so again if possible buy organic, preferably from an independent shopkeeper. It may be more expensive, but your body really is your temple. Also be aware of soya-based meat and diary alternatives such as, tofu, milk and yoghurt, as they may affect hormone balance. Take heed of the saying: *'Look after your body because it's the only place you have to live'* as it's true!

The pharmaceutical companies make billions of pounds by convincing us we need antibiotics, medicines, vaccines, over-the-counter drugs and a pill for every ailment known to man. All these drugs slow down our digestive system, may have avid side effects and make the manufacturers very rich indeed. I am not suggesting that you stop any medication that's been prescribed, but that you perhaps become more open to alternative, natural ways to medicate – make home-remedies, examine your stools and your tongue for any signs of irregularities and make the simple changes to your diet and lifestyle offered here in this book.

Health and cheerfulness naturally beget each other."
~ **Joseph Addison**

WHAT IS CLEANSING?

Detoxification for wellness purposes has become all the rage – even Oprah's at it with her *'21-Day Cleanse'*. The process itself is cleansing and nourishing the body from the inside out, so you not only look better on the outside, but feel better on the inside. It's not a case of starving yourself for a couple of days or even two weeks so you feel hungry and deprived – the objective is to clear the accumulated waste sensibly from the cells and tissues daily, so all the body's systems – circulatory, nervous, hormonal and lymphatic – run at optimum levels.

In this hurried world of fast foods, nicotine, alcohol and caffeine, our bodies have become overloaded and have trouble naturally eliminating this toxic material. Millions of people commonly suffer from irritable bowel syndrome, constipation and other digestive ailments.

Regular cleansing rids the intestines of parasites, the mucoid plaque that's accumulated on the inside walls of the intestines and other harmful bacteria so the body can operate in tip-top shape.

GETTING YOUR BODY ON YOUR SIDE

It's not difficult – your body is 100% on board with eliminating harmful waste at all times and better still, unsupervised. Most of it is broken down in your liver and then eliminated via the kidneys, colon, skin, lungs, nose and ears, so every time you urinate, exhale, cough, sweat, defacate and sneeze – you're detoxing!

With the premise that your body is attempting a full-body cleanse every minute of the day – the detox secrets that follow are not so much

> *Let food be thy medicine*
> *and medicine be thy food."*
> **~Hippocrates**

cleansing on their own, but more boosters to strengthen our amazing self-rejuvenating body. Think of them as motivational cheerleaders to encourage and support your body to rid itself of toxins.

This book is divided into chapters focusing on the body's primary detox organs: intestines, liver, kidneys, lungs and skin. In reality though, our body cleanses ALL of its cells and organs at pretty much the same pace – so an effort to cleanse any single one will have a positive effect on all the other organs, too.

Remember also that many symptoms of toxic buildup may have taken weeks, months or even many years to accumulate and cause problems. A twice-yearly seven-day cleanse will of course have a short-term effect, but the ultimate goal should be to embrace my idea of a Daily Detox to truly get the full benefit of your body's in-built anti-ageing, cleansing and weight-control system.

Physical and emotional rest, fresh air, water and decent nourishment are all you need to truly optimise cleansing and fully recover from toxic overload – time, as they say does heal all.

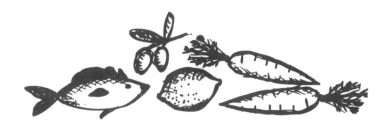

WHAT TO EXPECT WHILE DETOXING

Each time you introduce a new Daily Detox to your life, you may experience some symptoms, sensations, feelings and emotions – often different each time. The first few days or hours you may feel lethargic, nauseous, have headaches and your tongue may be covered in a white coating and in need of scraping.

On the other hand you may be absolutely fine! Also what you excavate and excrete may also be different too – so expect the unexpected and go with the flow, literally!

Remember – only you can tell what's best for you – listen to the subtle, neverending messages you get from your body and you won't go far wrong. I always say try everything – mix things up and yet be sensible – become more aware, be open to education and most of all, have fun!

THE TOXIN TALLY – HOW TOXIC AM I?

Give yourself a point for each 'yes' answer.

- ❏ Do you consume refined grain and flour products such as bread, pasta, white rice, cakes, breakfast cereals, cookies, crackers, snack bars?
- ❏ Do you eat non-organic vegetables, fruits or meat?
- ❏ Do you drink alcohol more than five times per week?
- ❏ Do you eat pasteurised dairy goods such as milk, cheese, yoghurt?
- ❏ Do you consume processed 'fast' food such as TV dinners, canned foods, candy, chocolate?
- ❏ Do you eat unfermented soy products such as tofu, soybean oil, soy milk, soy cheese, soy ice cream, soy yoghurt, soy 'meat', soy protein?
- ❏ Do you microwave food or beverages?
- ❏ Do you drink less than eight x 8-ounce glasses of water a day?
- ❏ Do you drink or cook with tap water?
- ❏ Do you drink more than four cups of coffee a day?
- ❏ Do you eat less than eight servings of fruits and vegetables a day?
- ❏ Do you have an office-based sedentary job?
- ❏ Do you use an electric blanket?
- ❏ Is there a powered electric device within 2 feet of your bed?

- ❑ Do you use a mobile phone next to your ear more than 15 minutes a day?
- ❑ Do you live in a city or near a major airport?
- ❑ Do you use non-natural chemical cleaning products and detergents?
- ❑ Do you use non-natural, chemical skincare and personal hygiene products?
- ❑ Do you take prescription, non-prescription or 'recreational' drugs such as antibiotics, antidepressants, birth control pills, HRT?
- ❑ Do you have skin problems or fungal infections such as acne, athletes foot, candida?
- ❑ Do you suffer from bloating, gas or indigestion following a meal?
- ❑ Do you have less than one bowel movement a day or get constipated occasionally?
- ❑ Do you smoke or are you exposed to smoke passively?
- ❑ Do you spend less than half an hour a day outdoors in natural light?
- ❑ Do you have root canals or amalgam 'silver' dental fillings?
- ❑ Do you sleep poorly? E.g. insufficient regular sleep, insomnia or disturbed sleep.
- ❑ Do you exercise less than three hours per week?
- ❑ Do you frequently travel by air?
- ❑ Are you overweight or do you have cellulite fat deposits?
- ❑ Do you feel tired, fatigued, or sluggish throughout the day?
- ❑ Do you suffer from 'brain fog' or difficulty concentrating or focusing?
- ❑ Do you have more than two colds or bouts of flu per year?
- ❑ Do you suffer from low moods or depression?
- ❑ Do you suffer with allergies, asthma, hay fever, breakouts, rashes or hives?
- ❑ Do you often suffer from physical or emotional stress?

TOXIN TALLY TOTAL

Now tally up your score to get an idea of the possible toxic load your body is dealing with.

25+ TOXIN TALLY POINTS: Oh dear, you're in the right place – your body is in need of some Daily Detox. You will certainly benefit from carrying out the suggestions in this book. Start with the *'easy'* ones first that you can change today and don't give up. Be honest with yourself, things seriously need to change even if you say you feel and look *'ok'*. Life has a way of letting us know we need to put our health first so heed any warning signs and immediately take action for a total body overhaul.

10-24 TOXIN TALLY POINTS: Not too bad – or *'could do better'* as they used to say in school. By focusing and taking your wellbeing seriously, even minor adjustments made to your diet, your exercising programme and your emotional and mental health will lift you out of that life-lull feeling, prevent premature ageing and prevent further gut upset.

0-9 TOXIN TALLY POINTS: Congrats, you are well on the way to enhanced longevity via a cleaner way of living. You take care of yourself already so keep up the good work. Fine-tune the areas that need attention and you'll be walking the talk, looking fantastic and leading a life full of health, vitality and wow.

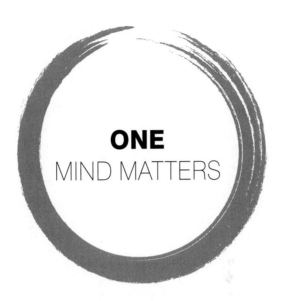

ONE
MIND MATTERS

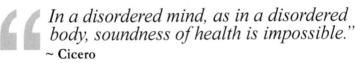

In a disordered mind, as in a disordered body, soundness of health is impossible."
~ **Cicero**

W hen most people think of detoxing, they usually think of cleaning out their bodies due to overeating, drinking too much alcohol, smoking or taking drugs. Many people detox to kick-start a weight-loss programme and this is perfectly fine; however, it's rather pointless to clear out the body's waste and reach an ideal weight when the mind remains in a state of chaos.

It's vital therefore to cleanse the mind/the brain/the head so we are clearer with our goals and more able to understand ourselves so we can change what we need to change. A clear head helps clear mind-fog, enhances focus, improves memory, brings mental and emotional clarity and when we're stress-free, our body's systems flow optimally.

When stressed and anxious, the body produces the hormone cortisol, and in excessive amounts, apart from causing premature ageing, it's been suggested that it's now the West's biggest killer and the underlying cause of the majority of illness and disease. Yes, of course sometimes life brings sadness and grief – a bereavement, a broken heart, loss of employment are by all accounts stressful situations – but by leading a healthy lifestyle, having a calm mind and being grounded, we are more able to deal with these situations like the clouds in the sky that come and go.

Our brain is a muscle and can be damaged by free radicals that cause oxidation and causes the brain cells to degenerate so you become forgetful and not able to concentrate as well. Our brain needs exercise – fun activities like dancing clear the cobwebs away so problems dissipate, and by trying out some of the suggestions here, apart from valuably increasing DHEA, the anti-ageing hormone, we will feel calmer, more chilled out, and enjoy enhanced longevity, with the risk of disease radically reduced.

01　THANK GOODNESS! / GRATITUDE

We are all human and not perfect. We have bad days, and can get cross, frustrated and downright angry. However, looking at life at a positive angle so we take stock of all the worthwhile things we have in our life – even on the days we think things can't get worse – will help us open our hearts and be more content and happy. Yes, there are certain situations, which may be incredibly sad or appear unfair, but these are often the times we learn the most, when we can evolve and move forward and which change us. Look a bit deeper and they can be very spiritual moments.

Practising gratitude helps us put life into perspective – so instead of wasting time complaining, being negative, gossiping or moaning, start to look for the positive in any situation – it is usually buried somewhere, even if you think it really isn't. The other day, sitting in a cafe with my dog, I became aware it was freezing cold in there and was going to complain, and then I noticed my dog was quite happy curled up on the floor and I was enjoying a delicious soup made by the cook who always makes me laugh, so instead of complaining, I put my hat and scarf back on and enjoyed my lunch. I know this is only a simple example to share and there are far more *'dire'* situations we may well find ourselves in. Practising gratitude makes us less anxious, less depressed and releases tension so we are not always demanding more or wanting something else. The mind and body becomes calmer, our inner workings are less stressed and our digestive system can work as it is designed to. Practising gratitude can also help you to feel less lonely, it lowers blood pressure and boosts our immune system.

Remember the sayings often expressed by our parents and teachers when we were kids – *'the best things in life are free'*, well we're adults now and we know they really are; *'the most important things are the things we can't count'*, so very true; and of course *'count your blessings'* – there really are so many things in life we can be grateful for. Why not start keeping a gratitude journal to count your blessings? Put every joyful moment on your list, no matter how small; celebrate special occasions like birthdays and anniversaries; give compliments and in turn accept them gracefully with thanks; smile and express gratitude to people in the service industries; enjoy special moments with friends and family; say thanks to your kids for helping around the house and even thank your dog or cat for teaching you unconditional love.

CLEANSE CLEVER

Download a gratitude app for your phone or tablet – some send you daily reminders and wonderful sayings to brighten your day.

02 **MIND MAGIC** / MINDFULNESS

Practising mindfulness gives magical results and is very *'in'* at the moment. Now often prescribed by Western doctors to ease depression, anxiety and to stabilise mood – lots of studies show it works. No need to sit in lotus pose though – mindfulness can be practised anywhere!

Take the time to *'notice'* – even if it's for only five minutes a day. Notice what you see, what you smell, the sounds you hear, what you are feeling and even what you are tasting in your mouth. Each time you do this, you strengthen your brain and boost the areas related to happiness and everyday wellbeing.

There are many books and websites where you can learn mindfulness. Consider taking a one-day taster session and if you resonate with it, take the full eight-week course – life will never be the same again! I first came across mindfulness whilst in St. Lucia and I encourage all my clients to give it a go – it can change your life.

CLEANSE CLEVER

To enhance decision-making and leadership, before you start your busy day at work, sit quietly in your office chair and take a moment to take a few deep breaths to become grounded and present. Feel your feet touching the ground, notice the parts of your body touching the chair and feel your clothes against your skin.

03 **LAUGH YOUR HEAD OFF** / LAUGHTER

A good ol' belly laugh not only works your abdominals, diaphragm and heart, it also releases endorphins, the health-enhancing hormones, into the body so negative emotions are released; you feel happier, less stressed and your immune system is given a well-deserved boost. It's said that children laugh about 400 times a day and by the time they become adults, it's dropped to a paltry 15 times a day!

Even if you don't feel like laughing, did you know faking it causes the same physical reactions as genuine laughter? I've certainly experienced false laughter leading on to a fit of giggles and along with it, a reduction in the levels of cortisol, automatically making me feel brighter and lighter.

Laughter creates such wonderful positive effects on our everyday wellbeing and having a sense of humour helps us take a more light-hearted view of challenging situations. Laughter is infectious, as is smiling, both helping you to connect positively to others. Remember the saying – *'you don't stop laughing because you grow old, you grow old because you stop laughing'*?

CLEANSE CLEVER

Watch comedies on TV or at the cinema, listen to entertaining panel shows on the radio, join a laughter yoga class and regularly surround yourself with the family and friends you love. Enjoy the cleansed and feeling of relief that laughter brings.

04 **GO OFF GRID** / DIGITAL DETOX

How sad it's got to the point that even at the dining table everyone is unhealthily addicted to checking their mobiles – we can't seem to get away from ring tones, text alerts and email dings. Even at a funeral I went to recently the congregation was reminded to switch off their phones! Consistently checking them raises stress levels. Social networking, although there are positives, has many negatives – lowering self-esteem due to constant comparison to others, and do you really need to know that Aunty Betty has just had her hair done?

Wifi and mobiles are absolutely everywhere and pretty much unavoidable and as us humans have been around for thousands of years, it's only in the last twenty or so that we have been subjected to this new surge of electromagnetic waves. Studies show we need to heed with extreme caution – these waves may negatively affect our health.

Choose when to have your phone on – if you need it for work, make a point of only activating it during working hours. At some places of employment, phones have to be kept in a locker so only turn it on during lunchtime and then again after work. Being on your mobile before bedtime interferes with sleep so keep calls to a minimum in the evening and turn off one hour before retiring. When in bed, leave your phone in another room.

Make a new rule to check emails only twice a day – say at 10am and again at 4pm. Have an automatic reply to incoming emails saying you only check at these times and only if it is urgent they can call you.

Spend less time online – although an amazing invention, don't get into the habit of needlessly Googling something. It really can wait and when checking genuinely for something, resist the temptation to go away from the subject in hand by checking social networks or playing games.

CLEANSE CLEVER
Seek out cafes, restaurants and theatres that have Wifi-free zones. Otherwise turn off your phone and be present with the company you are with.

05 **LET THERE BE LIGHT** / DAYLIGHT

Although we need to take care of our skin when exposed to sunlight, being outside during the daytime has enormous perks for the welfare of our mind by stimulating the production of the *'happy-hormone'*, serotonin – the body's all-natural and inbuilt antidepressant.

The sun also plays a crucial part in setting our sleep-wake internal clock by triggering the production of the *'wakey-wakey'* serotonin from sunrise to sunset and allowing its opposite, melatonin, to kick in at sundown, alerting us to prepare for sleep.

Unfortunately our present-day lifestyle completely disrupts our brain's need for unadulterated, unprotected sunlight. We don't spend enough hours outdoors and when we do, we are so covered and protected that it's useless to our brain. Artificial light outside of daylight hours totally bamboozles us into turmoil, sleepless nights and possible depression!

So if you feel down, get more daylight – draw back the curtains, roll up the blinds and let the sunshine pour into the house and get your workout gear on. Ditch the gym membership and work out outside – participate in your local park's boot camp class, power walk, join a running club, cycle, play tennis, take up golf – anything to get out in the fresh air, move your frame and clear your head.

Then when the sun goes down, use the dimmer switches, limit time looking at TVs, monitors, tablets, smartphones etc. and allow your mind to unwind and slip into an effortless restful sleep. You really won't believe the difference to your mood and how alert you'll feel throughout the day after making these basic tweaks to your lifestyle – it quite literally will be as different as night and day.

....

06 **BETTER OUT THAN IN** / EMOTIONS

We all feel better after a good cry and we feel liberated after we've danced our socks off – even though in both circumstances we may well be exhausted. *'It's better out than in'*, as I used to say to my kids when they were small.

Suppressing our emotions can lead to anxiety, depression and becoming bad-tempered, fearful and resentful. We may subconsciously distract ourselves by watching too much television, become addicted to sex, drinking or smoking in order not to face what we really need to address. Expressing our emotions (without the intent to hurt someone) is a way to clear our mind and reboot our energy levels so we live authentically, with openness and honesty.

If you feel pent up, writing down your feelings in a daily journal will help you release negative thoughts, and putting on your favourite tunes and dancing will discharge negative pressure.

Become creative and experiment with paint or clay or sand to express your feelings. And live life with a kind heart and healthy, open mind.

07 **FANCY CHANTS** / CHANTING

Chanting is one of the most beautiful ways to inner peace and a quietened mind. It's a wonderful way to relax after a busy working day or when your mind is chaotic. More and more yoga centres offer Kirtan sessions where you gather together to listen to the inspirational and spiritual sounds from India. Using a call and response method – the singer chants one line and you repeat it. I discovered the beauty of Kirtan on a trip to Ubud in Bali and now regularly attend sessions in London.

Buddhists practise chanting to prepare the mind for meditation and your local Buddhist centre will usually offer chanting classes. You don't need to attach any religious meaning to chanting and you can chant to any higher divine source or simply enjoy. I love sitting in a chanting circle and being with others as it offers a warm community feel. No need to be a soulful singer – I'm certainly not – and no experience is required!

Overtone chanting, a form of sound therapy from Mongolia, and described as a preventive medicine, has many mind and body advantages. Apart from relieving stress and tension, it may improve vision, ease headaches and even balance our chakras – the seven energy centres of the body. While a little more challenging to master, the sound is otherworldly – the combination of low notes with ethereal flute-like high notes just has to be experienced to be believed!

Chanting is true mind-medicine and an antidote to our hectic modern lives.

CLEANSE CLEVER

Often in yoga classes, we start and finish the session by chanting Om – this is pronounced 'aum'. Chant it anywhere and anytime to help you relax, bringing a sense of peace and serenity to mind, body and spirit.

08 **SWEET DREAMS** / SLEEP

S ound sleep is the best natural medicine there is – at night, whilst in slumber our internal organs and cells are working to produce extra protein to repair toxicity.

Sleep is essential to life – it affects everything to do with our day-to-day wellbeing and is the hallmark of optimal health. It's also the best antidote to the effects of ageing – our growth hormone levels shoot up at night, healing our skin and softening those dreaded lines. We need an uninterrupted bout of between six and eight hours with this *'silent healer'* each and every night – to reduce inflammation in our body, to reduce stress levels and to keep low moods out of our lives.

How many times have you heard the expression *'Oh you'll be much better after a good night's sleep'*? It's true – a disturbed night's sleep is a detox disaster – we wake up feeling grumpy and *'out of sorts'*, finding it difficult to concentrate and focus during the day – not to mention we're playing catch-up with those nasty toxins that have built up due inadequate time in slumber.

If you're having difficulty getting enough zzz's, try these super-slumber fixes.

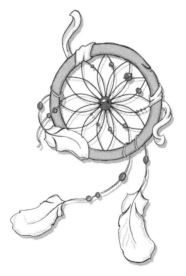

CONSISTENCY: Set a regular bedtime (preferably 10pm or before) and stick to it! Go to bed at the same time every night – even at the weekend.

CHILL-OUT: Set an hour of wind-down time before getting in to bed – dim all lights, switch off TVs and monitors – allow your brain to slip into sleep-mode.

EARLY: The zzz's before midnight are twice as valuable as the ones after – as the saying goes *'Early to bed and early to rise, makes a man healthy, wealthy, and wise.'*

DRINK: Resist drinking any beverages at least two hours before bed and restrict caffeine consumption to the hours before noon.

EXERCISE: Slot a bout of HIIT or dynamic yoga into your day.

ALARM: Rather than using a noisy alarm clock that shocks you out of sleep – train your natural internal alarm clock to wake you up just before the audible one – mentally repeat your desired time as you fall asleep.

OUTDOORS: Expose yourself to daylight to keep your sleep/awake cycle in tip-top condition – especially first thing in the morning.

ELECTRICS: Switch off all electric devices in or near your bedroom (especially Wifi devices and mobiles) – better still, ban all electrics from the bedroom.

COMFORT: Get comfy – room moderate to cool in temperature and a nice supportive mattress.

DARKNESS: Extinguish all unnatural light.

ALIGN: Sounds a bit off-the-wall I know, but try lying with your feet towards north – aligning with the earth's electromagnetic field.

BATH: Have a soothing Epsom salts bath in your wind-down time – the high magnesium content of the salts is a natural sedative.

Much underrated, napping has some seriously nourishing benefits too. It's a bit of a knack and the best time to give it a go is six hours after waking, and snoozing for no more than 15 minutes. When I was in Japan with my family, we were bemused at lunchtime when Japanese workers finished their meal, pushed their bowl out of the way and simply put their head down on the restaurant table to snooze! They napped for 10–15 minutes, woke up and went on their merry way – returning to work refreshed and revitalised – power-napping at its best!

Sleep to me is THE must-have ingredient for the perfect Daily Detox recipe.

CLEANSE CLEVER

Using blackout curtains really does help – any amount of light getting to your brain will trigger the 'gotta be awake now' response!

....

09 **DETOX DISASTER** / DIRTY DOZEN

The Dirty Dozen list is compiled annually by an environmental group that tests fruits and vegetables with the most pesticide residue – and although you can remove the peel on some of the fruits and veggies, you'll lose a lot of the goodness and nutrients by doing so.

Aim to buy organic or shop at farmers' markets, especially for the produce on this list. Or if you have outside space, grow your own. Although the government says pesticides are *'safe'*, there are many illnesses and diseases recorded by those exposed to them – cancers, dementia, birth defects, impaired fertility, and behavioural problems in children to name just a few. Pesticides are also detrimental to bee colonies and one of the possible reasons for colony collapse disorder – colonies of bees have simply disappeared. Be aware – pesticides are also carried in the air!

THE DIRTY DOZEN

✗ Apples
✗ Celery
✗ Cherry tomatoes
✗ Cucumbers
✗ Grapes (drink organic wine!)
✗ Hot peppers
✗ Nectarines
✗ Peaches
✗ Potatoes
✗ Spinach
✗ Strawberries
✗ Sweet bell peppers

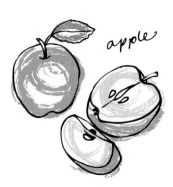

apple

CLEANSE CLEVER
Imported produce has the worst pesticide contamination – look for locally grown goods.

10 MAD AS A HATTER / MERCURY

Did you know that back in the 18th and 19th centuries, mercury was used in the making of felt and many hat makers slowly went mad due to the constant exposure to this very toxic substance? Mercury causes brain cell degeneration and there is strong evidence linking mercury to heart disease, Parkinson's, Alzheimer's, digestive problems, infertility, sleep disorders and kidney disease – the list is endless.

If you are of the generation that every time you visited the dentist as a child, a tooth was automatically filled with amalgam – then consider having them removed and replaced with composite white fillings. Amalgam has been used for dental fillings for over 100 years and is made up of half mercury and half silver and tin – it's the strongest, cheapest filling around and although the dental profession insists they are safe, low levels of mercury vapour are released into the body. Insist on white composite fillings no matter what your dentist says or – if you are in a financial position to – see an holistic dentist to have your old amalgam fillings removed and replaced.

CLEANSE CLEVER

Avoid heavy metal cleanses if you have mercury fillings – you'll only drag the toxic metal into your system and feel terrible – ditch the fillings first, then cleanse!

....

11 **AUNTY WHO?** / ANTIOXIDANTS

The body naturally produces damaging free radicals that cause oxidation and so in turn we need antioxidants to combat this damage and prevent diseases like cancer, Alzheimer's, deteriorating eye health and cardiovascular disease.

Although the body produces antioxidants naturally, our poor bodies just can't keep up the onslaught we inflict and we need more to bring about balance and harmony – also to combat the damage. My go-to antioxidant all-stars are: berries (blueberries, cranberries and blackberries), carrots, raw cacao, apples, prunes, walnuts, pineapples, all organic if you can find them.

Juicing a big bunch of kale and spinach every morning to make an antioxidant shot with attitude has become second nature to me now – it's quite an acquired taste so down it in one! Try adding ice to intense-tasting shots like this, it'll calm those sometimes overpowering flavours and adding lemon is a fab mixer too!

CLEANSE CLEVER

Because of the large variety of antioxidants that protect our tissues from different types of damage, it is best to include as many different antioxidant-rich foods as possible!

....

12 **HEAD START** / INDIAN HEAD MASSAGE

The ancient Ayurvedic art of Indian head massage works on the chakras of the body, our energy centres, clearing blockages and realigning these centres bringing, the body back into balance. Massage to the head stimulates blood flow, sending fresh oxygen and nutrients to the scalp, promoting new and stronger hair growth and by varying the pressure over the head, neck, upper back and shoulders, aches and pains are eased.

Different rhythms increase white blood cells, boosting the immune system and the efficiency of the lymphatic system to better remove fluids and swelling from the body. The face is also skilfully massaged ,leaving the skin glowing as facial muscles relax, lines are gently diffused and elasticity improves. Indian head massage is a relaxing way to release anxiousness, stimulate the parasympathetic nervous system, leaving you with a sense of peace and harmony, enhanced concentration and mental clarity.

CLEANSE CLEVER

Aches, pains or mild flu-like symptoms following a head massage are GOOD – your body's detox system is alive and kicking. Keep hydrated!

13 **HEAD OVER HEELS** / INVERSION THERAPY

Turn yourself upside down and feel the rejuvenating benefits of inversion therapy! Regularly practised by the US Army, it's a safe and effective way to recover from tough workouts, relieve stress and stimulate lymphatic circulation, speeding up the elimination of toxins. Often prescribed to reduce back and neck pain – hanging upside down elongates the spine, creates space between the vertebrae and relieves pressure on the discs. It realigns the spine into its natural S-curve, hydrating the discs, improving posture and alignment, and as we know, aligned posture helps you look younger and more elegant.

Invest in an inversion table or attend aerial yoga classes where you practise yoga poses hanging in a hammock (made out of material similar to that used for parachutes). I do a class once a week with my daughter – it's terrific. Hanging upside down also increases oxygen to the brain so concentration and memory is enhanced, headaches are decreased and balance is improved. You'll also notice flexibility increases, varicose veins are eased and you'll literally feel space between your joints.

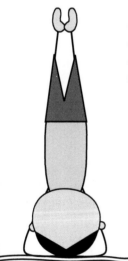

Inversion therapy is a wonderful way to re-energise after a busy day at work – and although a slightly different take on yoga, headstands, shoulder stands and handstands offer very similar perks!

CLEANSE CLEVER

As 'King of the Yoga Poses', standing on your head not only reverses gravity, but claims to reverse ageing too – try it and see the world from a more youthful and awakened angle!

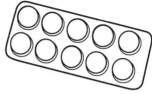

14 **BAD PHARMA** / MEDICATIONS

t's not only illegal drugs that are poisoning our bodies, but legal, prescriptive and over-the-counter (OTC) medications too – simply peruse the shelves full of different pills, potions and painkillers for all the various type of headaches, coughs, colds and aching joints we are supposed to have. Some of these drugs are highly addictive and most of them have severe side effects – some causing hallucinations, liver failure, stomach problems, suicidal thoughts and even death.

Legal drugs also include birth control pills, HRT, thyroid regulators, pills for high cholesterol, antibiotics and statins for blood pressure. There's a pill now for virtually every ailment and desire. Need help on a diet? Swallow a slimming pill. Must have bigger muscles? Down a muscle-enhancer. Want to make your friends laugh? Inhale a dash of helium! And if you need to rise to the occasion and stay there then simply pop a Bluey. The list is endless. Legal drugs are as dangerous to our prosperity and wellbeing as illegal substances – staying in our gut affecting our good bacteria, disrupting our digestion, mood and personality.

We are well aware of the most commonly socially accepted drugs – alcohol and nicotine – which are progressively and rapidly addictive, but there are also millions of people unfortunately dependent or addicted to painkillers and sleeping pills. If you are addicted, start by confiding in someone you trust and seek professional advice to help you get clean. Support groups have lots of success in helping you beat your addiction and the guidance of an holistic doctor will support you through your detox cleanse.

15 FAT CHANCE! / GOOD FATS

Change your thinking and ensure you include fats in your diet – good fats that is! Avoid low-fat, reduced-calorie and fat-free commercial produce as the missing fat is usually replaced with sugars, refined carbohydrates, salt and additives and is partly responsible for the West growing fatter in the last 20 years. Trans fats are also guilty parties to this increased weight gain, unhealthy cholesterol levels, increase in depression, hormonal problems and premature ageing. Bad fats also promote free radicals affecting our long-term welfare.

Our brain is made up of about 60% fat and we need healthy fats in our diet. Saturated, monounsaturated and small amounts of polyunsaturated fats contain omega-3 and omega-6 essential fatty acids. These increase blood flow to the brain, helps to slow cognitive impairment and even help maintain a healthy weight. Flax seeds, wheatgerm, sunflower seeds and pumpkin seeds are all rich in omega-3, so include them in your recipes.

Consumption of oily fish has drastically reduced over the last century so many of us are way off balance. Include wild salmon, mackerel and sardines in your diet at least three times a week for optimal brain power and a healthy nervous system. Notice also how the appearance of your skin improves and you'll also feel less anxious and tired.

Cut out those low-fat spreads immediately and use butter instead – yep, good ol' grass-fed unsalted butter. Stop buying low-cal salad dressings and make your own using olive oil, avocado oil or Argan oil. Resist the temptation to buy cheap fatty meats, hamburgers, cookies, breakfast cereals, crisps, pizzas and ready-prepared meals no matter how much the kids beg – and fill your shopping basket with lots of walnuts, hazelnuts, pecans, Brazil nuts and macadamia nuts as snacks. Nuts are superb, rich sources of good fats that will not only keep those sugar cravings at bay and your waist trimmer, but also greatly sharpen the mind to make you feel younger and at the top of your game!

CLEANSE CLEVER

Coconut oil is my versatile fat friend – I discovered this whilst in Hawaii way back when. Can be used in cooking, added to smoothies, great as a hair conditioner and a natural glistening, all over body moisturiser.

16 **MENTAL MOVES** / MIND FITNESS

As the saying goes, *'if you don't use it, you lose it'* – and that can be applied to lots of different situations – from working out and enjoying sex, to exercising the brain.

Doing a crossword every day or solving the puzzles in your daily newspaper will keep you sharp and alert, improve your focus and enhance concentration. Crosswords increase vocabulary as well as trivia knowledge and you may well become healthily addicted! Find the simple pleasure and satisfaction in brain teasers, word finder and word challenge puzzles and notice your speed and progress. Get rid of brain-fog by playing board games like Scrabble and Trivial Pursuit – a social way to connect with family and friends – or join a group to meet new people and learn bridge or poker.

Learn a new language – when we travel abroad why do we expect everyone to speak English? Even picking up words and phrases helps us be more on the ball and it's a warm feeling when we are understood. Is there an instrument you learned as a child and would like to resume? I learned the piano until I was about sixteen and then *'teenage life'* got in the way, but I've started lessons again now and although rusty, I'm determined to re-master *Für Elise* and *Dizzy Fingers*!

Take up writing – spend ten minutes a day writing a journal or just scribble down your thoughts and feelings. Join a creative writing class to help you finally write that novel – be brave, set your inner artist free and unleash your innate urge to create something different. You never know, you could be the next J. K. Rowling!

We all know about the mind-body connection so keeping the body healthy means keeping the mind and the brain healthy too – physical activity sends fresh blood flow to the brain to improve alertness, memory and attitude. I have an adorable lady of 86 who comes to my yoga class every week – an inspiration to me because of her cheerful and positive outlook and attitude to life.

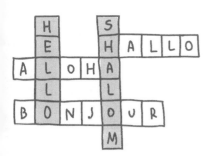

CLEANSE CLEVER
Supercharge your brainpower by learning something NEW – regular use is of course a must, but the challenge and sometimes discomfort of LEARNING and being in foreign waters is the killer ingredient.

17 **PLAIN & SIMPLE** / DECLUTTER

Do you find you have *'stuff'* around the house just in case you need it or that the dining table has to be cleared each time before you can use it? Many of us have a tendency to keep things we no longer need or have boxes we mean to sort through, but if your clutter starts to cross over into hoarding and have a negative effect on your wellbeing and your family's life, then it's a problem that can escalate if not kept in check. Compulsive hoarding is a psychological disorders that requires professional help.

Most of us may be a little bit guilty of having a rather full wardrobe of clothes, or an untidy desk, so let's remember the saying a *'clutter-free house means a clutter-free mind'*. We all know that one person's idea of disorganisation may be someone else's chaos; however, take a careful look around your house and honestly assess the mess!

Put a date in your diary to clean out each room. Enjoy the feeling of liberation and satisfaction once it's done – it really is refreshing. Start with the wardrobes – if you haven't worn outfits or shoes in the last two years, be brutal and get rid of them – either to a charity of your choice or sell them on eBay.

Us girls know that make-up drawers and bags and bathroom cabinets often contain a multitude of mascaras, lipsticks, and nail varnishes we never use – be ruthless and chuck out what you no longer need. It really is quite easy when you get into the swing. I helped a friend recently sort out her make-up and she had a blusher compact from when she was 16. She's now 44!

Clear your kitchen cupboards of old utensils and broken crockery and out-of-date jars and all cans. Avoid falling for supermarket marketing *'buy one get one free'* offers, *'3 for 2'*, or the latest must-buy that week – it's all a ploy to get us to spend more on even more stuff we don't need! And don't forget to clear out under the sink – safely dispose of chemical cleaning fluids, air fresheners and dish-washing powders and replace with eco-friendly items.

Engage the whole family in the clear-out. It teaches everyone to be respectful of each other's space and it teaches decision-making skills. If you find it too stressful deciding whether to chuck or keep, then do a little at a time. It can be overwhelming sometimes, so avoid the stress and continue the next day. I know a friend who found her clearing-out decisions a whole lot easier after she picked her favourite dog charity to donate the goodies to.

CLEANSE CLEVER

When trimming down the medicine cabinet, return out-of-date medications to the local pharmacy rather than throwing them down the toilet and further polluting our water! Restock with essential oils, homeopathic medicines and apple cider vinegar (ACV) – an excellent anti-fungal!

18 TALK TO THE HAND / TOXIC PEOPLE

Become selective who you spend your precious time with and notice if you feel drained after being with certain friends. If so, just as you declutter your house, declutter these people! Accept the way they are – you cannot change them – and realise there are toxic folk out there and they have no place in your life – even if they've been around a very long time. Obviously I am not suggesting you desert a friend you care for deeply when going through difficult times. We all have people we love even if they drive us a bit nuts sometimes! You'll always be there for each other through life's ups and downs.

Surround yourself with interesting people, those who make you laugh and those who want the best for you. It's damaging to our physical and mental states hanging out with manipulators who we feel obliged to see, or who only want to see us to talk about themselves. Go with your gut instinct – if spending time with someone is heavy and enduring or you don't feel good about yourself and feel consistently criticised or judged, then maybe have a conversation with them about how you feel. They may be going through things in their life they haven't shared so be grown up and try to see their point of view. However, as we know, no one can make us feel anything without our permission and I'm sure we all know people who insist they are always right and we are wrong. Be honest and kind to yourself – and with them – and let them go. Cut ties before any more destruction is done!

If you're working with someone you find irritating, ask for a transfer of department if possible, or change your job (maybe not so easy in today's employment market).

If that's not viable, change your perspective on the situation and look to learn from it. It usually teaches us acceptance, patience and forgiveness in some way (which doesn't mean allowing yourself to be mistreated in any way). I once worked in a team where we felt our manager didn't lead by example – one rule for her and one rule for everyone else – it irritated us all. However, after she became pregnant, she softened and was a delight to work with – she'd been trying for years to conceive and had been going through her own private hell.

As we get to know ourselves better, it becomes easier to pick up on negative energy from others, and even though sometimes it's not always easy to let go of these flawed relationships – we have to empty our cup to make space for new, beautiful and exciting people to enter our lives.

CLEANSE CLEVER

To enhance your sense of adventure, hang out with adventurous people who welcome situations out of their comfort zone. Challenging situations improve confidence and raise self-esteem.

19 COMING UP ROSES / *RHODIOLA ROSEA*

f you're feeling in a low mood, the *Rhodiola* plant can help you get your bounce and wahoo back! Studies have shown it raises serotonin levels – the happy neurotransmitter that sends messages to the nervous system so we feel right with the world and energy levels are elevated. We also feel more motivated and positive about life.

Rhodiola is named after the rose-like scent of its roots and has been used for centuries for physical and mental endurance and enhanced performance – it also lowers cortisol levels, which in excessive amounts can make us feel overwhelmed, disturbs our blood sugar levels and cause gut problems.

It's an unlikely place to find the scent of roses, but *Rhodiola* can only be found natively in the most inhospitable climates of the far north, like Siberia. Gladly however, it's available in a capsule or as a tea (a dandy choice), making it ridiculously simple to take advantage of one of nature's brain-boosting and anti-ageing goodies!

CLEANSE CLEVER

Avoid taking right before bedtime, as it may interfer with sleep.

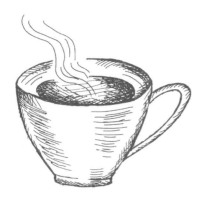

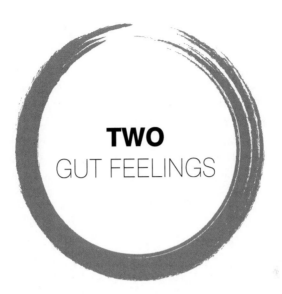

TWO
GUT FEELINGS

Your gut is always right."
~ **Sharon Osbourne**

Our small intestine is where food digestion continues after leaving our stomach. Nutrients are extracted through the intestinal wall and taken into our bloodstream to be transported to wherever they are needed. The waste then moves into our large intestine a.k.a. our colon where water is re-absorbed and waste is prepared to leave our body.

When waste moves too slowly or builds up, toxins are reabsorbed into the bloodstream, gradually making us feel ill. In an ideal world, we should move our bowels after every meal – just like a baby – but we're lucky if we eliminate once a day! For many, constipation is an accepted way of life, but this is most certainly not a healthy condition.

Even if we eliminate regularly, two or three times a day, our colon can still become toxic over time. Waste matter can accumulate and continuously release poisons back into the body.

Another way the colon becomes toxic is from our poor dietary habits – so even though transit time is *'normal'*, certain foods and additives are toxic to the body, and when absorbed slowly poison our cells, muscles, nerves and glands. Inevitably disease and illness follows. It's not uncommon for an adult to accumulate 10-20 pounds of toxic waste, and King Henry VIII of England was reported to have 84 pounds of waste matter in his bowel when he died!

The design of the modern toilet (by plumber Thomas Crapper) has not helped facilitate evacuation of the colon. To empty the colon we were designed to squat. So squatting by raising our feet up on a footstool of about 12 inches high or thereabouts in front of the toilet is recommended. And practising squats when you work out will certainly aid fluid digestion, ease constipation and ensure full elimination.

Gut cleansing is in my option THE most important area to focus on when considering a whole body detox system. Below are some wonderfully soothing and rejuvenating tonics to help keep you feeling youthful and beautiful – on the inside.

....

20 **BARE BONES** / BONE BROTH

More and more we are moving back to simple, traditional foods and cooking methods our great grandparents would have been proud of. Numerous cultures worldwide have a recipe along the lines of: Toss the remains (bones, skin, fat, meat i.e. the lot) from last night's chicken dinner into a pot with a few veggies, cover with water, season and simmer for the whole day – et voilà – chicken soup or bone broth.

I do admit though this simple recipe doesn't hold much culinary sex appeal, however to Michelin-starred chefs the world over, it is the basis of their fine cuisine, and after perusing the ridiculous healthy benefits it holds, you too will see it in a different light.

The magic ingredient comes in the form of collagen, a much craved and publicised ingredient in the beauty world, and bones are packed with the stuff! During the slow, long cooking process, the collagen breaks down into gelatine and in this we find the REAL *'secret sauce'* – amino acids, specifically arginine, glycine, proline and glutamine. Our body struggles to produce adequate amounts of these when we're sick or under stress, and considering most people's baseline of health, our body is screaming out for these aminos most of the time!

The killer benefits of these awesome aminos really do stack up – protection for the gut lining, cellulite reduction, regeneration of damaged liver cells, a stronger immune system and better wound healing. They are also needed to make the super-antioxidant glutathione, help detox the body of chemicals and finally help heal leaky gut syndrome.

The high levels of calcium, magnesium and phosphorus make bone broth a nutrient-rich and sometimes free medicinal food with superfood status that should be on everyone's menu who wants effortless youthful skin and superstar digestive health!

CLEANSE CLEVER

Add a couple of tablespoons of apple cider vinegar to your broth recipe – this acts like a sponge, pulling out even more minerals and nutrients from the bones during the cooking process!

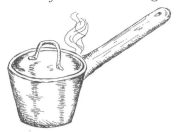

21 **A BIT OF ROUGHAGE!** / FIBRE

Dietary fibre is one of the unsung cleansing heroes of our digestive health, a bit like the gut highway patrol and totally essential for excellent belly health. It keeps food and waste traffic flowing freely with minimum transit time, as well as maintaining even blood sugar levels and dealing with poor driving conditions like yeast and fungus build-up too.

The gut highway patrol comes wearing two different uniforms: soluble and insoluble. The soluble cops slow the speed at which food is digested, keeping you full for longer which is appropriate for weight loss and blood sugar balance and the insoluble fibre cops work at higher speeds, passing though the gut quickly, preventing infections and toxic build-up through constipation.

It's not so important to worry about getting the balance of the two fibres right as Mother Nature does that, and by eating plenty of fresh fruit and vegetables in your diet, you will be well on your way.

My top five friendly fibre foods are – broccoli, cabbage, berries, leafy greens and celery.

GREEN SOLUBLE SMOOTHIE

Ingredients:

Spinach / 2 cups
Mint / 1 handful
Coriander / 1 handful
Mango / 1 small
Celery / 4 medium ribs
Fresh ginger / ¾–1 inch or to taste (peeled)
Lemon / 1 tbsp juice

Directions:

Combine all the ingredients in high-speed blender. Add a little water at a time if needed to thin the blend.

CLEANSE CLEVER

As juicing removes nearly all the fibre, it can potentially cause problems with blood sugar levels, especially if you are juicing mainly fruits. Lean more toward green juices — as these have minimal effect on blood sugar.

....

22 **THE WHOLE PICTURE** / ORGANIC FOOD

What actually does *'going organic'* mean to our day-to-day living? Eating as cleanly as possible is top of my list when it comes to reducing the toxic load on the body as food and drink are by far the biggest source of nasties our detox organs have to deal with on a daily basis.

Sourcing whole organic food can take a little time though, so firstly swap over the not-so-good choices on an *'as you find it'* basis. Next check out the Dirty Dozen list (p. 37) to identify the most toxic fruit and vegetables and find replacements for these. Then visit the local whole-food store and farmers' market as this opens a vast network to tap into in order to make the transition.

I find the biggest challenge to making organic meal choices is eating out in restaurants or gatherings with friends and family. More restaurants though are becoming conscious of their diners' desires and this is reflected on the menus. Friends and family are used to what some consider my strange ideas of healthy, and don't mind and even welcome the contributions when I answer their inquisitions!

Sometimes however, there will be no perfect options, so go with the flow, it really is OK. I operate on the 90:10 rule – 90% of the time I follow my organic is optimal mantra and the other 10% there's no guilt or mind games – have that piece of non-organic apple pie!

CLEANSE CLEVER

When cooking, avoid undoing all the organic goodness by over charring on the barbecue or denaturing in the microwave.

....

23 **ALIVE & KICKING** / PROBIOTICS

Believe it or not, 1.5kg of our body weight is actually made up of a vital population of 100 trillion bacteria inhabiting our gut, and without them we would be unable to neutralise harmful toxins or maintain a strong immune system. This detox army living in our intestines is made up of good and bad bacteria, which is pretty dandy so long as they are balanced. Think of it like weeds in the garden – you can live with some, but left untended they will take over and ruin everything. Getting the balance right is really quite simple – eat up your prebiotics and probiotics!

Prebiotics are the foods we eat that feed the good bacteria, helping them to multiply and crowd out the bad ones, found in all the foods containing soluble fibre. Probiotic foods on the other hand actually have the good bacteria within them, so by eating them you're boosting the ranks of the friendly bacteria.

Fermented foods such as miso, raw apple cider vinegar, sauerkraut, kombucha, kefir and yoghurt are all packed with friendly, living bacteria, ready and willing to help with detoxing and cleansing the body.

....

24 **CHEW IT OVER** / CHEW YOUR FOOD

Digestion isn't simply what happens in our stomach and gut, it starts way before we even lay our eyes on food! We've all had conversations about what we're cooking or eating for dinner later, ending with feelings of hunger and our mouths watering. The water is actually highly alkalising saliva packed with digestive juices and is the body getting ready for the main event – eating a meal – and digestion starts immediately in the mouth as we start chewing.

Having the mouth water before eating anything is vital to effortless digestion and if it's not, you need to ask yourself if you are actually hungry or if that particular food is the best choice for you right now. If the answer is a big ol' *'No'* – you're only inviting some unwelcome guests to your dining table – indigestion and bloating.

The simple solution is to take a mindful eating approach to dining. Switch off your chattering mind (and chattering mobile!) and consciously eat and appreciate your meal. If possible, eat in silence and take a few moments to truly connect with the food you are about to consume. Think about how it will taste, appreciate its colour, allow your anticipation to grow and digestive enzymes to build, ready for action.

Once food is in the mouth, savour the flavours and textures, chew a few more times than you would normally so the solid food leaves your mouth as a liquid – as Mahatma Ghandi said *'drink your food and chew your drink'*.

Mindful eating is super on many levels, it's destressing for mind and body, stimulates great digestion, inhibits overeating and helps you maintain a healthy weight.

....

25 **SWEET NOTHINGS** / SUGAR DETOX

Our sweet tooth not only leads us to obesity but also causes serious inflammation in the cells of our body. Due to it being so highly addictive, we daily gobble down huge volumes of the stuff – a massive 22 teaspoons a day on average! So forget the sweet dreams as not only does sugar cause insomnia, but is also linked to an ever-growing list of health problems including hair loss, skin conditions, tooth decay, hypertension, depression, allergies, colon cancer, heart disease and diabetes. So, a bit of a problem then!

Shunning the toxic white stuff by way of clean eating is probably the easiest way around the problem. Processed foods are sugar-laden, even the foods not considered to be outwardly sweet have hidden sugars, including ketchup, pasta sauces, salad dressings and mayonnaise. Be wary of low-fat labels too, peel off that label and you'll find a high-sugar one hidden beneath!

26 **IN MINT CONDITION** / MINT

Spearmint and peppermint – I love them both, the scent alone is so rousing and refreshing. As a digestive tonic, both have been A-listers since the Roman times, with their healing powers widely documented and prescribed for all sorts of digestive upsets and detoxification.

Although different plants with similar tastes, peppermint may be a tad stronger and its medicinal properties come from the menthol it contains. Spearmint being milder may be more suitable for children and cooking and its taste comes from a property called carvone.

When I think of either – a nice cup of cleansing tea comes to mind, particularly beneficial after a meal to aid quiet digestion and can also relieve acid reflux. Or chew on a few leaves to freshen breath or bundle some stems together with a band and pop them into your restorative bath. Peppermint oil applied topically on the temples will ease headaches, or as a decongestant, a few drops on a tissue does the trick. A glass of warm water with some spearmint leaves is said to halt hiccups and is also brilliant for flatulence – although I don't think at the same time, but you never know!

My green Mighty Mint juice below is a fabulous digestive aid and detoxifier.

MIGHTY MINT JUICE

Ingredients:

Mint / a good handful
Lemon / ½
Green apple / 1 crunchy variety
Cucumber / 1 medium

Directions:

Push all items through the juicer in the order above. Give it a swirling swoosh around in your mouth to get the full fresh and zesty effect.

CLEANSE CLEVER
Pop a few drops of peppermint oil onto a handkerchief before an important meeting or exam – clears the mind, improves memory and enhances focus!

27 HOT-TO-TROT / CAYENNE PEPPER

Chilli is my go-to spice when I want some heat and zest in my food, and cayenne pepper is from this fiery family. It's the hot captain in my spice rack.

While not for the faint-hearted, when adding it to your favourite curry dish, cayenne has been on the wellbeing and cleansing scene for a very long time – used in Traditional Chinese Medicine (TCM) for thousands of years and popular in Ayurvedic medicine too. It's anti-inflammatory, lowers blood sugar, boosts circulation, reduces gas and bloating and helps with stomach acid production to improve digestion, reducing the toxic load in the body.

Cayenne is a powerful antioxidant as it's full of flavonoids, brilliant for anti-ageing and also a solid source of vitamins C, B6 and E. Its main active ingredient is capsaicin, which relieves tired muscles, aching joints and arthritis. Yet, don't restrict its spiciness to savoury dishes – add a dash into your freshly squeezed green juice or yummy green smoothie recipe. And one of my favourite uses – added to chocolate desserts! By the way, research shows it can also aid weight loss – pretty useful after that moreish chocolate dish!

....

28 **BOTTOMS UP** / OIL ENEMA

Most of you reading this will be well aware of the therapeutic benefits of enemas and colon hydrotherapy, and yet unaware that as well as being a primary elimination exit, the colon can also absorb nutrients. A basic enema is inserting water into the colon via the rectum. The ancient Indian art of Ayurvedic uses oil, called *'basti'* to nourish and detox the colon. It also uses probiotic supplements, bone broth, ghee, sesame oil, raw honey and herbs – the list of possible combinations is quite extensive and somewhat surprising!

In comparison to a traditional water enema, the volume used for a basti is greatly reduced (¼–½ cup) and the hold time may be up to half an hour or longer. Whereas a normal enema focuses on the eliminative action of the colon, the yogic version cleans much further, acting as a therapy to purify and pull toxins from all over the body.

Don't be fooled by the small volume though, the basti ingredients have a profound effect on the body and can be a challenge to retain for even 5 minutes.

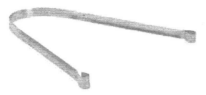

29 **TONGUE-LASHING** / TONGUE SCRAPING

Considering our tongue takes up half the space in our mouth and is also in one of our main detox exits, few of us pay it much attention. The age-old Indian art of Ayurveda however recognised its significance and came up with the idea of scraping the tongue daily to improve cleansing and oral hygiene. The painless and easy process is best done first thing in the morning and in less than ten seconds eliminates that ugly white coating of bacteria that can lead to bad breath.

As well as being a fantastic cleaning tool for tongue and mouth, the process of scraping also increases our awareness of tongue hygiene – the amount of build-up, the colour and tenderness while scraping. In the Ayurvedic system, tongue health is actually a reflection of what is going on in other parts of the body – similar to reflexology – the most notable being gut wellbeing, so a furry tongue could mean excessive toxins in the digestive tract, leading to poor digestion and associated problems.

I was initially a bit unsure of the idea when a friend told me about tongue scraping, but you only need try it once to enjoy the clean, fresh feeling in your mouth afterwards. Follow this with your morning teeth routine and you simply can't go wrong – such quick and effective mouth magic!

CLEANSE CLEVER
When choosing a tongue scraper, go for stainless steel rather than toxin-ridden plastic.

30 **SMOOTH OPERATOR** / FLAX SEEDS

As usual, good ol' reliable nature has created a small and perfectly formed, superfood – the flaxseed (a.k.a. linseed) – and the phrase good things come in small packages couldn't be more true here. Rich in both soluble and insoluble fibre as well as antioxidants and the beneficial omega-3 essential fatty acid (EFA), the flaxseed has been blessed with many detoxification powers. Although our prime focus here is on gut health, studies suggest that the little seed can protect against cancers of the breast and prostrate as well as the colon.

Ground flaxseed is my secret ingredient when making smoothies as the high EFA and fibre content do a fantastic job of balancing blood sugar levels when eating fruit smoothies. Or sprinkle some over your salad to help ease constipation.

GO WITH THE FLOW SMOOTHIE

Ingredients:

Oranges / 1 cup freshly squeezed juice
Strawberries / 1 cup (fresh or frozen)
Banana / 1 medium (frozen)
Ground flaxseed / 1½ tbsp
Coconut oil / 1 tbsp

Directions:

Blend the ingredients together and enjoy your yummy hit of good fats and fibre – cayenne is fantastic in this too if you like a bit of heat.

CLEANSE CLEVER

Don't be bamboozled by a name: milled, ground or flax meal – they're all the same!

31 **AGAINST THE GRAIN** / GLUTEN FREE

Since when did eating whole grains lead to such toxic turmoil? If grains are indeed so bad for our bodies, how come we've been eating them for more than 10,000 years? Well, in that time grains have changed, and it's like playing with an innocent and cute month-old baby and then 14 or so years later being reunited having not seen each other in between – would we even be able to recognise the teenager?

Grains have grown up too, with wheat changing the most from its infant state, and sadly, its evolution has been far from natural! We as humans have had a huge influence in its development, especially in the past 50 to 100 years. We've genetically modified it to produce higher yields of grain and sprayed it with pesticides and herbicides to further enhance production volume. Then a whole slew of chemicals, additives, enhancers, enzymes and trans fats are added before it reaches our mouths – in short, we've created a *'frankenfood'*!

Bottom line: grains are not designed by nature to be digested, they actually contain compounds that actively fight digestion and this is a problem for the gut. The most problematic substance being a protein called gluten, derived from the Latin word for GLUE! Having a sticky protein in our intestines over a period of time is disastrous and causes inflammation and toxic stress.

I've found my clients who've cut grains from their diet for a few weeks are astounded by their improved sense of wellbeing and health. Everyone can benefit from a reduction in products containing grains (pasta, bread and breakfast cereals) and your gut will be first in line to congratulate you on the decision.

....

32 **BELLY BLISS** / ABDOMINAL MASSAGE

Abdominal massage is an awesome therapy for detoxing and toning the gut, and it's something you can easily do yourself! Your main focus is on the colon, which begins at the bottom-right of the abdomen, moves up and across below the ribs and then back down to the bottom-left of your tum. The movement is a continuous clockwise flow of one hand over the other using a gentle pressure at first. Areas that feel a little more tender than others can signal congestion in that part of the colon so performing small circular movements in that area will generally do the trick and get things moving.

Also try different positions while doing the massage – most people find lying on their back to be the easiest position in which to relax and get mind-blowing results. Drawing the knees up and dropping them to the sides, can also create different angles to help reach those hard-to-get to spots. Sitting on a stool is another option to experiment with and I find using a little coconut oil helps keep the movements flowing and soothing.

Finding what works for your particular biology is the real art of belly massage, but once you get the hang of it, the rewards of a calm and effective colon cannot be understated – toxins are eliminated swiftly, weight loss is a breeze and you will have youthful and radiant skin.

33 **BOUNCING ALONG** / REBOUNDING

Although a far cry from the bouncy branch of gymnastics we call trampolining, the humble rebounder or mini-trampette can be included as a cleanse friend with a winning reputation.

It's anti-ageing efforts are insanely good and its design is pretty much unchanged from its debut back in the 70s. Its fitness advantages are huge – conditioning for the heart and lungs, better balance and co-ordination, low impact (so less strain on the joints) and it improves lymph circulation leading to better full body detoxification. Finally, it enhances digestion and elimination. You'll be bouncing off to the toilet in no time!

Rebounding is also fool-proof for those HIIT sessions – simply alternate between all-out bursts and short recovery periods for a total time of 10-15 minutes. Be mindful of your breathing though, it can be tough work. Aim to include at least one of these fun bounce sessions in your workout week and jump up and down to your fave tunes. Twisting targets the abdominals and those love-handles!

CLEANSE CLEVER

If you're new to rebounding, you don't even need to jump up and down, simply bending and straightening the knees is beneficial.

....

34 **WORTH ITS METAL** / ZINC

We all know oysters perk up the libido as they are plentiful in zinc, a powerful mineral that helps maintain a healthy reproductive system and a high sperm count in males. Gobble up what's on the platter and throw in some zinc-filled lobster on the side and those little tadpoles will soon be swimming in the right direction in no time!

Did you know though that zinc is a powerful antioxidant and is found in every tissue of the body? It isn't just beneficial for sexy nookie sessions, but is also a valuable essential trace element for the gut, stimulating over 100 enzymes in the body and aiding smooth digestion, easing diarrhoea, IBS and leaky gut syndrome (yep, not as glam as having a good ol' romp but still pretty useful for our gut).

Zinc sources don't need to be extravagant, raw cacao does the same trick and so do cashews and pumpkin seeds. Try this bad-ass smoothie below with zinc galore!

THINK ZINC SMOOTHIE

Ingredients:

Raw cashews / ¼ cup
Water / ¾ cup
Pumpkin seeds / 1 handful
Raw cacao / ½ tbsp
Banana / ½ small
Raw honey / 1½ tbsp
Wheatgerm / ½ tbsp
Extra virgin coconut oil / ½ tbsp

Directions:

Create a milk base by blending the cashews (pre-soaked for 6 hours if you have time), pumpkin seeds and water. Add in the remaining items and blend until smooth. Drink and feel your zinc levels rise and your gut send gratitude!

CLEANSE CLEVER
As well as being a liver tonic, garlic has ample levels of zinc.

35 BAN THE CAN! / NO CANNED FOOD

Pretty simple really – avoid eating canned foods. I know it's easy and quick to open a can of something when we're hungry – a soup, or throwing canned peas in to some dish – but adopting the habit of blanching fresh organic vegetables and making hearty homemade soups is far healthier for the brain and our bodies.

People who eat canned food regularly are shown to have a higher level of bisphenol A (BPA) in their urine when tested. BPA is a by-product of the chemical that prevents can corrosion and can lead to liver dysfunction, cardiovascular disease and diabetes. Remember to ditch the canned drinks as well and buy water in glass bottles instead.

George Orwell was pretty spot on when he said: *'We may find in the long run that tinned food is a deadlier weapon than the machine-gun'* and I stand by my mantra of *'Ban the Can'*!

CLEANSE CLEVER

Ditching a habit that isn't serving you is all about researching and finding substitutes – wise words from Benjamin Franklin: 'If you fail to plan, you are planning to fail!'

....

36 THE FAST LANE / INTERMITTENT FASTING

We've all experienced that desire to just switch off from day-in, day-out stresses that can lead to emotional and physical exhaustion if left unchecked – even a single-day trip to a wellness spa can be enough to help rejuvenate us. Our gut too yearns for a break from a similar day-in, day-out stress that we constantly subject it to – the huge volume of low-nutrient food that needs to be digested and eliminated. We could actually be wasting up to 10% of our vital energy in an effort to keep up – maybe more if we are going heavy on the junk food!

Our busy lives and long working hours add to this burden by encouraging us to start eating breakfast early on in the day, then constant snacking and at least two other main meals – it isn't uncommon for people to eat their final meal between 9pm and 10pm in the evening (later on the Continent). It's no wonder our gut is miserable with this state of affairs – it is constantly under attack while we're awake and getting less than eight hours sleep is completely rubbing salt into the wound!

Sometimes when our body's cries for moderation go unnoticed, it has to resort to desperate measures – it goes into super-detox mode leading to such weakness that we become bedridden, with food the last thing on our minds. Cleaning up our diet of course can help avert this enforced downtime, but reducing the sheer volume of food and upping the amount of time spent fasting, is the real game-changer here. That's where intermittent fasting (IF) comes to the rescue – in its simplest form, it is stretching the fasting time in between our last meal in the evening and first meal the next morning.

The 5:2 Diet, popularised by Michael Mosley, is a form of IF – five *'normal'* eating days, and two days of restricted calorie intake, that's 500 calories for women and 600 for men. The system has lots of inbuilt flexibility too – choose days that suit you best, they don't even have to be back-to-back and timing of the *'eating window'* is completely up to you.

Intermittent fasting is a fantastic strategy to have in your detox and weight loss toolkit, and even though eating an hour earlier in the evening and an hour later in the morning appears a tiny change to your routine, your gut will tell you otherwise. Try it for yourself – you won't be disappointed!

CLEANSE CLEVER

If you're choosing the low-calorie option select foods with lots of good fats – this keeps our blood sugar even for effortless fasting.

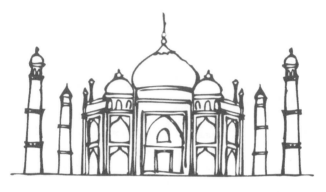

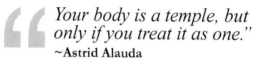

Your body is a temple, but only if you treat it as one."
~Astrid Alauda

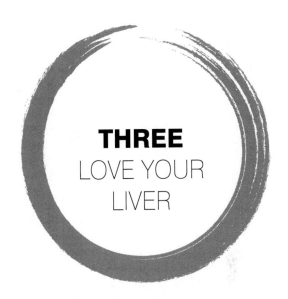

THREE
LOVE YOUR LIVER

" *Old age is when the liver spots show through your gloves.*"
~ **Phyllis Diller**

The body's second-largest organ (the skin being first), the liver, is made up of four lobes and is found just below the diaphragm, overlying the gall bladder. It weighs about three pounds – the body's heaviest organ – and is the major organ for detoxification.

Everything ingested passes through the liver so it's a tough little worker. It produces about one litre of bile each day to aid fat digestion, it stores glucose for energy and plays a major role in metabolism.

Too much bad fatty food, artificial sweeteners, an overload of sugar, an indulgence in alcohol and caffeine addiction all cause the liver to swell so you feel bloated, constipated, heady and bogged down. Many people's liver works only at around 40% of its potential capacity and when this organ is sluggish it can result in yellowing whites of the eyes, dark circles under the eyes and sallow skin. There may also be abdomen pain, darkened urine, acid reflux, fluid retention and chronic fatigue. Liver problems are also a contributing symptom to Parkinson's and Alzheimer's.

Under the right conditions, however, did you know the liver can regenerate itself within 6 weeks? These tips will help the liver heal and repair itself so it functions supremely and it can do its detoxifying job with pride. And as a little sideline – the word liver derives from the old English word for *'life'*!

37 ON THE RISE / KUNDALINI YOGA

Fifteen years ago, all I knew about Kundalini yoga was that it enabled *'something'* to rise within me – and then once I started to practise this style of yoga more regularly when in Sydney, the more I appreciated its amazingly profound healing benefits. That *'something'* is the energy that lies dormant at the base of the spine. Through physical postures, chanting and breathing techniques, the energy rises up the spine to the pineal gland, strengthening your whole body and restoring your mind, filling you full of love, grace and kindness.

Practising Kundalini also offers amazing support for the liver. A clogged liver may affect libido, mess with your menstrual cycle, bring on early menopause and leave you feeling out of balance.

Here's a super-duper sequence for detoxifying the liver (and get a six-pack at the same time, so can't be bad!):

- ❈ Lay flat on your back and extend your legs along the ground.

- ❈ Place your hands, palms downwards, underneath your buttocks to protect your back. Inhale and raise the legs to 60 degrees holding your breath for as long as comfortable, even if it's only a few seconds at first.

- Then as you exhale, draw the knees in towards the chest. Inhale again and extend the legs out one more time to 60 degrees and retain the breath.

- This time as you exhale, lower the legs carefully to the ground.

- Repeat the sequence two more times.

Be mindful when working with breath retention, you need to work gently and gradually build up your capacity to 15 seconds. Apart from rejuvenating your liver, you'll also be looking pretty sexy on the beach!

CLEANSE CLEVER

Kundalini yoga is a one-stop detox programme – including pranayama, chanting and dynamic yoga stretching.

38 CLEANSE CHIEF OF STAFF / GLUTATHIONE

'Cleanse Chief of Staff' or referred to by some as the body's *'master-antioxidant'*, glutathione is certainly THE buzzword when talking detox, anti-ageing and weight loss. Many studies show low glutathione levels is linked to everything from autoimmune problems to cardiovascular disease.

The master-antioxidant is THE most critical and integral leader of our detoxification system. It rounds up all free radical toxins and escorts them swiftly to the colon and bladder to be ejected from the body. Glutathione is then recycled and leaps back in to action and all is good. A problem arises, however, when our toxic burden is too much and levels drop to leave us open to illness and premature ageing.

Although oral supplementation of glutathione has proven largely ineffective, there are ways to nudge our body in the right direction to up production by itself. Here are my seven killer effective and natural glutathione boosters.

1. Eat **sulphur rich foods** such as garlic.

2. Eat **grass-fed dairy** – raw milk and eggs.

3. **Exercise** regularly – try HIIT or rebounding.

4. Eat **grass-fed red** meat and organ meats.

5. Add **turmeric** to your diet.

6. Reduce stress in your life – **mindfulness, laughter** and **breath awareness**.

7. Supplement with **milk thistle** (p. 87).

CLEANSE CLEVER

The lowest levels of glutathione are found in the elderly – so as we age boosting our glutathione levels should be THE number one anti-ageing goal.

39 **CLEAN SWEEP** / LEMONS

Since singer Beyoncé dropped weight big time using the Lemon Master Cleanse known as the Lemonade Diet, developed way back in the 1940s, it's regained huge popularity. It's a cheap way to detox, however, if using it to specifically drop weight, beware. Such strict dieting on the lemon juice with maple syrup and cayenne pepper, along with the herbal laxative teas and salt water drinks suggested may well leave you feeling hungry and moody with loss of lean muscle tone to your body – especially after the recommended 10 days! You will lose weight for sure but watch out, it may go straight back on if you're not careful.

Lemons, however, are a brilliant liver detoxifier and flush out built-up waste and prevent gallstones. Although an acid-tasting fruit, when ingested, they alkalise the body and balance pH levels. Start the worthwhile digestive habit of drinking a glass of warm water and lemon every morning as it wakes the digestive system and aids peristalsis and freshens morning breath. It's a diuretic and is said to improve weight loss. Lemons have been used since the ancient times to combat infection – it's an antibacterial and antiviral fruit and we've all heard of a cup of warm water, lemon juice and honey to fight off colds and flu. It's amazing for the skin too, topically applied, it can clear spots and blackheads leaving skin clear and flawless and if you're unfortunate enough to be stung by a bee – just apply lemon juice! If you fancy your hair a shade lighter in the summer time, adding it to your final rinse after shampooing, naturally lightens your strands.

CLEANSE CLEVER

To eradicate the smell of fish from your hands after handling, scrub with lemon and adding slices of lemon and lemon juice to fish whilst cooking, exterminates that awful smell from the whole house.

40 **UP BEET!** / BEETS

Back in Roman times the Gladiators ate beets to maintain sexual vim and vigour. This deep purple root contains lots of boron and increases the release of nitrate oxide into the body, which sends blood to the genitals, so no Viagra needed back in that day then!

Ages ago too, the Indians also found it useful for counteracting anaemia as they knew beets are full of vitamins, iron, potassium and magnesium, helping relieve fatigue and lethargy, regenerating the red blood cells. My ancestors, the Greeks, meanwhile offered it up on a silver platter to Apollo the god of the sun and music.

Today a silver platter is not needed and beets are best eaten raw – they do wonders for supporting the cleansing process, protecting bile ducts and healing the kidneys in the process. Beets get their colour from the antioxidant betacyanin that brightens the complexion so it becomes smooth and clear, and it also diffuses wrinkles.

For a liver cleanse detox booster, create a green juice that includes beets AND their green leaves – the leaves contain even more iron than spinach – or grate raw beets on top of a salad to add colour and vitality.

CLEANSE CLEVER

Eating beets may turn you urine and stools pink! No need to panic.

....

41 **REFLEX ACTION** / REFLEXOLOGY

I know in the West it can be difficult to get our head around the fact that certain parts of our feet correspond to certain parts of our body – but they really do. Reflexology involves a specialised practitioner pressing trigger zones of the foot with varying pressures to balance the nervous system and increase circulatory and lymphatic movement enabling fresh oxygen and nutrients to be delivered to the cells. This speeds up the elimination of waste from the heart, liver and kidneys.

Reflexology clears blockages and stagnation along the energy meridians of the body so energy can flow freely, so you feel more relaxed, destressed and re-energised. The practitioner, with your feedback, works on reflex points to balance the kidneys, the bladder and the gut.

You can also '*do*' reflexology on yourself – there are no negative side-effects even if you don't get the exact point – it may be tender, quite painful and yet all positive! Standing on a shakti mat is another option – you'll definitely *'get the point'* here!

In my Pilates class, I ask my clients to place one hand on the wall for balance as they place one foot on a tennis ball, pressing down mindfully to find those 'tender' points.

42 JUICE IT UP / GREEN JUICE

By having one green juice a day you can fortify your liver to ensure it's carrying out its vital health-sustaining duties of supporting the digestive system, regulating fat stores and controlling blood sugar levels, thus restoring balance, serenity and harmony to the body.

Regular juicing is a nutritious and safe method to cleanse the accumulated toxins from the intestines, and having a nutrient-dense and alkalising juice every day is an achievable challenge for most of us. Avoid convenience – store-bought juices are usually made from concentrate, are high in sugar and full of ugly additives and preservatives. It really is far better to create your own green juices at home using fresh vegetables and fruit – all organic, of course.

Investing in a decent juicer is the first place to start. I first got into juicing after watching *'Fat, Sick and Nearly Dead'* where an overweight Joe Cross with his many ailments cured himself after 60 consecutive days of juicing. His experience has since inspired thousands of people – not just to cure themselves of their varying illnesses, but has motivated the fit and healthy to juice daily at home as part of a lifestyle choice. Even my son (who is very aware of how he looks in the gym and on the beach) is now in the habit of having a fresh green juice each morning before work.

Daily Juice Challenge

To help you with the *'Green Juice A Day'* challenge I've created seven juices to kick-start your cleansing journey. You'll find these on page 145.

> CLEANSE CLEVER
> *If you're a newbie to these highly nutrient-dense green juices – it can be quite a shock to your stomach – diluting with water will ease the shock and help your body cope massively.*

43 CHEERS! / ALCOHOL

Excessive alcohol inflames and scars your liver and causes cell destruction – it's as simple as that! Over-board drinking causes a fatty liver and the liver is under such severe strain it simply cannot do its health-promoting job. Continue to drink in such an excessive way and bang – you're dead – (even though it may take a few years!). Alcohol accelerates the loss of brain cells, impairing memory and judgement.

It's worrying to think the increase of alcoholic liver disease has gone up by 30% in the last decade and the average age has decreased as more and more younger people's drinking gets out of hand. Alcoholic liver disease accounts for 2.5 million deaths worldwide each year and it's a fact that one in four drinkers with fatty liver disease develops hepatitis with one in five developing cirrhosis.

Ideally, for the happiness of your liver – avoid alcohol completely. Experiment with other drinks – I like water with a squeeze of lime or iced green tea with crushed ice in an elegant wine glass, or try a virgin cocktail of cranberry juice with mint.

For the wine drinkers out there, you'll be pleased to know there are more and more studies that suggest having a quarter of a glass of good red wine a day (half a unit) protects the heart and prevents cardiovascular disease, raising good cholesterol levels. Red wine contains resveratrol, a powerful antioxidant that helps prevent oxidative damage, which causes premature ageing and degenerative conditions.

I'm certainly not advocating you take up drinking – yet when out with friends for dinner, and if you fancy, maybe have a small glass then. Bear in mind though – over the last few years, wine glasses in bars and restaurants, along with the measures, have sneakily increased to the detriment of our health and waistlines but not their profits!

CLEANSE CLEVER

If you are drinking alcohol every day, consider having a few alcohol-free days every week so the liver can have some reprieve. If you think you may have a problem with excessive drinking and would like help, don't delay and consult your doctor.

....

44 **VAMP IT UP!** / GARLIC

Eating lots of garlic may ward off vampires and be useful in the Twilight Zone; however, this little unassuming bulb, part of the allium family, does wonders to clean the liver and help prevent constipation.

Known as one of nature's wonder drugs, garlic is rich in sulphur, a mineral that helps the liver get rid of waste by activating liver enzymes, improving its bile production and regulating liver fat storage. This superfood helps expel toxins from the body more efficiently. If you can live with the after-whiff, eat raw for optimal healthy liver function, a strong heart and efficient circulatory systems.

As an antibiotic, these powerful cloves are unsurpassed, being shown to be more potent than penicillin and yet without any interference to that vital balance of our gut bacteria that penicillin has. It contains anti-inflammatory properties too, so is also useful for skin conditions such as psoriasis and athlete's foot and the presence of allicin and selenium protect and prevent the liver from toxic damage. Another sulphur-rich superfood for liver detoxification, is garlic's modest cousin, the onion – from the same family and helps regulate blood sugar levels and an ace ally in the fight against free radicals.

Parsley is a perfect partner to garlic and onions to help counterbalance their, considered by some, unsociable effects. Make this simple dressing to harness the literal *'killer'* effects for your immune and detoxification system.

PARSLEY PESTO DRESSING

Ingredients:

Raw cashew nuts / ½ cup
Organic extra virgin olive oil / ¾ cup
Fresh parsley / 1 cup
Fresh basil / ½ cup
Garlic / 2 cloves, finely chopped
Salt / ½ tsp
Cayenne pepper / to taste (optional)

Directions:

Begin by grinding the cashews to a powder. Blend the cashew powder and all the other ingredients. Now slowly add water – testing as you go – until you reach the desired consistency.

....

45 **FOOLISH FATS** / TRANS FATS

Yep there are foolish fats – and rather foolish behaviour when we scoff trans fats, a.k.a. trans fatty acids, a.k.a. partially hydrogenated oils (PHO) – created by the industrial process of adding hydrogen to a naturally liquid vegetable oil to create something much thicker or even solid. Unfortunately when these *'frankenfats'* are introduced to our body, they no longer speak its natural language and are sent packing to the nearest exit – adding to the toxic load our liver has to deal with.

Cheap to make and used a lot in restaurants for commercial frying, found in fast foods, margarine spreads, cookies, pastries, pizzas – (the list is endless) – trans fat may add life to produce shelf life – but shorten our life! Trans fats overwork the liver, build up plaque in the arteries and lead to heart attacks and heart disease.

A type of trans fat also occurs in trace amounts naturally (very importantly) in some meats too, like lamb and beef – these are in such small amounts and because of their natural origins, our body understands what to do with them and can effortlessly process them through our system.

Trans fats are just a complete detox disaster and should be avoided like the plague, simple as that – getting them out of your life will be a game-changer and your longevity and detoxification will skyrocket. No excuses please!

....

46 **SOUR SAVVY** / APPLE CIDER VINEGAR

Cold-pressed organic raw apple cider vinegar contains lots of valuable natural minerals and vitamins and its unique acids help the body eliminate toxins more efficiently, fighting bacteria, parasites and yeast. It regulates cholesterol levels, reduces heartburn and helps the body achieve balanced acid/alkaline levels.

Take a tip from our Eastern friends and use ACV (as it's known), for detoxification of the liver and improve the body's circulatory system. Unprocessed, unpasteurised and unfiltered, Mother Nature's *'miracle'* contains lots of living enzymes to add good bacteria to the gut. Studies have shown that adding a teaspoon to a glass of water and sipping eight glasses throughout the day aids weight loss (obviously not whilst consuming hamburgers and apple pie!) and adding a cup to your bath water provides relief for sunburn. Don't worry, you won't smell of vinegar – it has a pleasant apple aroma.

Avoid using cheap ACV, which has virtually no redeeming qualities but lots of artificial colourings instead. ACV has a multitude of uses, from removing teeth stains to one of your eco-friendly kitchen cleaning products.

47 **BITTER & TWISTED** / BITTER GREENS

Go on, be a dare devil in your choice of greens and choose flavoursome bitter and dark varieties. In Traditional Chinese Medicine (TCM), dark bitter greens are prescribed to stimulate the liver chi (energy) and assist in the detox process, easing stagnation and congestion.

By choosing chickweed, stinging nettles, dandelion leaves, watercress or rocket – all rich in vitamins A and E and beta-carotene, production of saliva increases and improves digestive function by increasing gastric acid secretion.

Blanching the leaves releases the nutrients and dressed with a small amount of organic olive oil and Himalayan pink salt makes the leaves taste even more delicious. Mustard and turnip greens are the most bitter and have been shown to help prevent cancer and try broccoli, collards, endive or radicchio as a change from popular spinach, lettuce or kale, giving an extra boost of vitamin K, calcium and fibre.

CLEANSE CLEVER
Traditional Chinese Medicine (TCM) promotes the idea of eating more bitter greens to help ease sugar cravings – a detox win-win for sure.

....

48 **RAW DEAL** / RAW FOOD

Raw foods contain living enzymes that naturally fight our bad bacteria and strongly alkalises our body. When we cook our food these enzymes get destroyed and the nutrient value of vitamins and minerals are drastically reduced. Eating raw foods helps us stay grounded and connected to Mother Nature – you'll find you have more stamina, be more alert and sleep better.

All mammals eat their food raw and it's only us humans who actually cook our food, so it's rather interesting to note that not many of us will actually die of natural causes as they do in the animal world. Mammals live up to eight times their maturation age whereas we humans, just four times our maturation age!

When eating raw foods, you'll feel more alive with increased energy and vitality and more focus – nature provides a completely faultless menu option: balanced pH, packed with digestive enzymes, and high in friendly fibre. Think of how strong those beautiful gorillas are – and they only eat raw plant food, guided by their natural instinct and not by colourful recipe books.

Eating lots of raw organic fresh vegetables and fruits is cleansing and purifying for the whole body, not just the liver and gallbladder, and offers us all the nutrients we need for a greater sense of wellbeing. Unfortunately we live in a fast-moving real world of caring for the family, paying bills, working, going out with friends and generally having a full life – but with a small shift of mindset it's pretty straightforward to up the raw food portion of your meals to 80%. And raw doesn't just have to mean just chopped up vegetables and fruit, you can make green smoothies and fresh green juice too.

CLEANSE CLEVER
Choose spring or summer to start upping your percentage of raw food – your body will be naturally drawn to nature's light and nutrient dense bounty in these seasons.

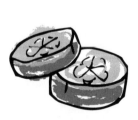
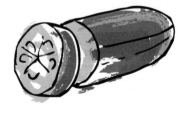

49 **FEELING FULL YET?**/ EMOTIONAL EATING

Most people eat too much! Either from not being mindful enough or using food as emotional comfort. Too much food – even if it is the most nutritious organic creative presentation out there – is harmful to our digestive system, our waistline and our minds.

Were you brought up with food being used as a reward? Did you have to eat everything on your plate before you could have dessert? I can't tell you the amount of times I've heard people say they *'deserve this muffin'* as their reward for working out. I even heard Arnold Schwarzenegger say in an interview the other day: *"The first thing I did when I arrived in London was to hit the gym and then follow that up with a delicious English dessert!"*

When you were small, did you eat to please, eating everything up because you were told to and feel guilty if you couldn't? And maybe as a child when upset you were comforted by a warm drink and biscuit rather than being listened to. Lots of things in our past are the basis of how we view and treat food today. We often eat from our heads rather than from our belly.

If you're someone who starts a diet every Monday, then a stressful day at work means you binge to feel better, momentarily do, and then feel disgusted with yourself – you're caught up in a vicious circle. You feel there's no point in losing weight, so continue eating, under a cloud of unhappiness and a growing waistband.

Emotional eating is eating to fill emotional needs and not the belly. However, it's not just negative emotions that can cause overeating but positive ones too! Feeling happy may mean we eat more and when out socially enjoying the company of friends, we may tend to continue eating and drinking long after we are full.

Combat emotional overeating by taking a moment or two before you grab second helpings or that extra biscuit and ask yourself if you really need it. If you are still hungry or searching to fill a gap somewhere else – be honest with yourself. Eating mindfully, slowly and with intention will help you consume *'proper'* size portions for your body. However, if your problems with food are more serious and deep-rooted, then seeking professional help and joining a support group will help you combat the addiction.

CLEANSE CLEVER

If you're eating due to boredom – call a friend and get out in the sunlight and fresh air for a HIIT session – exercise first, eat later!

....

50 **A STATE OF MIND** / MEDITATION

The media have pretty much put it out there that practising meditation is advantageous for mind and body. And they're spot on. The emotional and physical perks are well documented – it brings about a deep sense of peace and calm, reduces tension and anxiety, eases aches and pains, lowers high blood pressure and is anti-ageing – the list goes on. Did you know though, it's also beneficial for digestive health and optimal liver function? Who would have thought that sitting quietly in lotus pose can help our intestinal tract and aid liver detoxification? Many detox retreats and programmes include daily meditation as an important practice to reduce stress and acid levels and it plays a huge part in cooling the liver, easing congestion and stagnation and switching on the parasympathetic nervous system.

To ease the imbalances of the liver, (no need for lotus if that's not your thing), simply sit comfortably in a chair or lay down on your back to practise this specific liver meditation I discovered whilst on a retreat in India a few years ago.

Place your hands just under the ribs on the right side where the liver is and take a few moments to focus on the breath – slowly and deeply inhaling, slowly and fully exhaling. Then on the inhale, gently begin to massage in a circular direction anti-clockwise using the palms of your hands as you visualise cool, fresh spring water flowing into the liver nourishing and replenishing it. As you exhale, visualise the excessive heat, the stagnation, frustration and congestion all releasing from the liver. Continue for five to ten minutes. Now rest the hands on the lower abdomen below the naval and enter a state of thoughtless awareness and peace.

Our liver is an amazingly capable organ – it is strong and powerful.

CLEANSE CLEVER

There are different types of meditation and it's best to try a variety to find a style that resonates. If it's a challenge to practise on your own, start with just five minutes sitting quietly twice a day, gradually increasing the length of time to 20 minutes. Or join a local group or class at your nearest yoga studio.

....

51 **DISH THE DIRT** / EDIBLE CLAY

You won't go far wrong by looking to nature for the low-down on how to fire-up your body's inbuilt detoxification routine – take look at one way animals get rid of toxins – they eat dirt and clay!

Many animals including birds, gorillas, chimpanzees, rats, cattle and bats regularly consume mineral-rich clay. Even today, many native peoples across the globe still enjoy eating clay on a very consistent basis. And why on earth would they do this?

Well, many of the minerals essential for optimal health are pretty much dirt or rock when you get down to it – salt being the most obvious example. But acting as aids to detoxification is where these clays really become superstars. The canny animals and indigenous people subconsciously know that the clay acts as a toxin magnet as it moves through the digestive tract – attracting all the trash and flushing it out of the body.

There are several varieties of edible clays available from online health food stores – my favourites are bentonite clay and zeolite. Both are fantastic cleansers and immensely beneficial as part of our daily detox efforts.

Zeolite is a mineral compound found naturally in volcanic rock and bentonite is a clay created from aged volcanic ash with varying concentrations of several minerals including potassium, sodium and calcium. There are numerous scientific studies that show using zeolite during detoxing helps remove mercury from the body as well as arsenic, lead and cadmium. These heavy metals have been shown to be a contributory factor to Alzheimer's disease, dementia and some cancers.

One teaspoon of these clays, mixed with water or in your favourite breakfast green juice, can help get your bowel function back to normal, knock allergy symptoms on the head, boost your immune system, alkalise your body, banish free radicals, and best of all, lessen the burden on your liver.

CLEANSE CLEVER

Add a couple to tablespoons of zeolite or bentonite to you bath for a kick-ass detoxification soak!

··

52 **TO THE BITTER END** / DANDELION ROOT

Sulphur-rich dandelion root helps promote bile formation (due to its bitter taste), restores tone to the digestive tract and eases

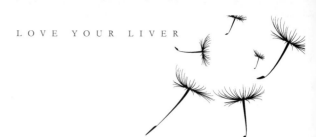

arthritis, gout and constipation, as well as being an efficient colon cleanser. Due to its high potassium levels, dandelion root is mildly diuretic, removing excess water from the body and inducing the flow of gastric juices. It eases constipation and improves poor digestion.

Drinking two cups of caffeine-free black and bitter dandelion root coffee every day is a healthy alternative to your usual latte and a powerful liver cleanser to boot.

We can all do with a little extra liver support as our livers (and lives!) are often over burdened with not only high trans fat diets, alcohol and bad pharma, but car exhaust fumes, chemical household cleaners and other toxins – so a cup of dandelion root espresso acts like your liver's guardian angel as well as easing bloating, inflammation and gas. And as a bonus, your skin will look smooth, youthful and flawless.

CLEANSE CLEVER

Remember it's not just the root that's a detox delight – the bitter leaves are also elite cleansers – just half a dozen leaves in your green juice, salad or green smoothie will have your liver jumping for joy.

....

53 **SILLY BUM!** / MILK THISTLE

Take the morning after the night before! Milk thistle is a medicinal plant which has been used for centuries for calming the liver after a heavy night out and a friend of mine swears by it. Known scientifically by the name of *Silybum Marianum* – I love that name – it's a safe option to ease liver-related diseases, including alcoholic cirrhosis, fatty liver disease and chronic and active hepatitis. Milk thistle is part of the aster plant family, which includes daisies, artichokes and thistles – and gets its name from the milky white fluid extracted when the leaves are crushed.

Lots of studies show the numerous benefits of milk thistle to improve bile function and ease spleen disorders, and it lowers bad cholesterol levels and regulates blood sugar levels.

Milk thistle is a powerful antioxidant, protecting the body from free radical damage and lipid peroxidation and has shown to have anti-ageing properties too. Pass me the *Silybum* please!

CLEANSE CLEVER

Do NOT self-medicate for any condition with milk thistle; talk to your medical professional first as it can interfere with other medications.

....

54 **CALM & COLLECTED** / CASTOR OIL PACK

Edgar Cacey was an American healer at the turn of the century who invented the castor oil pack to heal and soothe gall bladder and liver disorders. Calming, relaxing and soothing, do every night when cleansing your gall bladder, easing liver disorders and promoting sound sleep.

Here's the way I suggest: Take a large organic cotton flannel and saturate it in a bowl of cold-pressed castor oil. Have a hot water bottle at the ready and two towels. Place one of the towels over the couch or your bed for protection and lay on your back. You can have a bolster under your knees for extra comfort.

Now place the oily flannel directly on the abdomen, just on the bottom of your ribs and ensure the right side of the stomach is covered. Now place a bio-plastic bag over the flannel and place the hot water bottle on top of the bag. I suggest you wear some old shorts and midriff top in case you get oil marks over your clothes. Cover yourself snugly with the second towel and relax for at least half an hour.

To remove the castor oil pack, first take away the top towel, hold onto the water bottle and sit up. Place the towel over your lap and slowly remove the hot water and allow the flannel with the plastic bag to drop onto your lap. Fold the towel, bag and flannel in half together for use again. Massage the remaining oil into your belly in a circular clockwise direction.

CLEANSE CLEVER

Regular use of a castor oil pack over the liver has also shown to improve eye health and reduce eye puffiness.

55 **SOME LIKE IT HOT** / SAUNA

The Finnish gave us the sauna – which literally translated means *'sweating bath'* – a dry heat that works on the same principles of inducing sweat for purification like the Turkish baths (or the steam room at the gym). The Romans had the thermal baths, the Russians had the *'banya'* and the Japanese, the *'onsen'*. In fact most cultures have their own type of sweat bath or have adopted the sauna or steam room for detoxing. And although the sweat room is today thought more of a luxury rather than a necessity, aim to visit at least once a day whilst detoxing to speed up the regeneration of new cells, prevent premature ageing, aid weight loss and ease mental fatigue. Heat and sweat do wonders for boosting serotonin and endorphin levels and have a calming yet energising effect on our mental and physical state.

Sitting quietly in the sauna, (usually heated by rocks), for at least 30 minutes will naturally get rid of waste and inner impurities through the pores of the skin, and remember, the skin is the biggest organ in the body. Sweating promotes the production of white blood cells and boosts the immune system, and we all know the old-fashioned remedy for a cold is to sweat it out, as heat and sweat help neutralise the body's viruses and bacteria.

CLEANSE CLEVER

After the sauna, be brave enough to jump under a cold shower to shock the body and stimulate the circulatory systems to further speed up the elimination process.

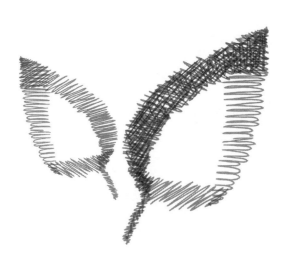

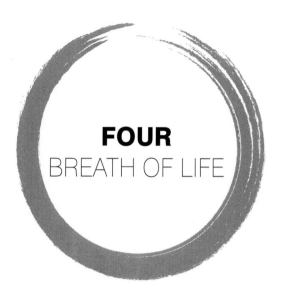

FOUR
BREATH OF LIFE

Breathe. Let go. And remind yourself that this very moment is the only one you know you have for sure."
~ **Oprah Winfrey**

Every time we inhale, our lungs absorb life-giving energy from the air in the form of oxygen, and as we exhale we release toxins and waste products from various metabolic processes back into the atmosphere in the form of carbon dioxide. While resting we perform this cycle around 12 to 20 times a minute, consuming around 11,000 litres of air every day.

Amazingly, 70% of waste is eliminated through the lungs, but sadly as a consequence of low air quality due to mould, dust, chemicals, second hand cigarette smoke and car exhaust fumes, again only to name a few, our lungs are completely overburdened and in need of some TLC – tender lung care.

When the efficiency of our lungs is reduced, the flow of blood carrying wastes from the kidneys and lungs slows too and our lymphatic system, which fights off viral and bacterial invaders, is weakened and our digestion may falter – not good!

It's no wonder we suffer from shortness of breath, coughing, poor circulation and congestion. However as you will see, simple dietary, exercise and lifestyle choices can have profound effects and have you breathing easy in no time!

....

56 **LUNG LIBERATION** / NICOTINE

Pretty obvious in my book – free your lungs and just say no! Nicotine addiction kills someone somewhere in the world every 15 minutes and smoking is the most preventable cause of death. It can be a stimulant, a relaxant and a sedative, producing free radicals in the lungs and then circulating around every part of the body – to all the organs, narrowing the arteries and raising blood pressure. It increases the likelihood of strokes, cancer, heart disease and causes countless other chronic diseases. It reaches the brain in approximately 15 seconds – and kills the brain cells! It affects outer appearance too – premature ageing, wrinkles around the mouth yellow teeth, grey skin, dull hair and how you smell!

Secondary smoke is also very toxic – although most of the toxins have been inhaled by the smoker – it's still not much fun being in the same room – so if it's a situation where you're unable to leave, ask them politely to go outside and do their puffing. And by the way, did you know that pets also die sooner if their owners smoke?

Nicotine is one of the hardest addictions to give up. So reduce situations where you would naturally have a puff – give up coffee, wine, beer and drink antioxidant-rich green tea instead.

Eating organic liver and more oily fish, which are rich in vitamin A, helps protect the lungs and as smoking makes the body more acidic, eat lots of fruits, veggies, wheatgerm and buckwheat to bring the body back to a healthier alkaline state.

Hypnosis has been proved to be effective in helping smokers to stop, as has support by various quit-smoking charities, and of course, seek advice from your doctor too. Gain the support of your family and friends and consider asking other quitters how they succeeded.

CLEANSE CLEVER

Each time you would have bought a pack of cigarettes, save this money in a piggy bank – you'll be surprised how much you will have collected and treat yourself to a spa day!

....

57 LOVELY LUNGS / SWIMMING

We've all heard how swimming is one of the best forms of exercising and it's right up there at the top of my lung detox list. Superb for all ages, all shapes and sizes, easy on the joints, terrific for rehab and best of all, it's fun.

Think of the fine definition of a swimmer's body – swimming increases muscle strength and tone, improves flexibility and importantly it strengthens the heart so it can pump efficiently, enhancing blood flow and breathing efficiency. Swimming has also shown to help with asthma problems, increases lung capacity and even reduces snoring!

It's worth investing in swimming lessons to improve technique and alignment – how many of us swim badly with our head out of the water to keep our hair dry? Spinal alignment and correct breath control is important when swimming so we not only swim elegantly and gracefully but our body and lungs are boosting optimal capacity from each stroke.

Participating in weekly aquatic aerobic classes is a brilliant way to improve cardiovascular fitness – jumping up and down, running on the spot, kicks and swaying side to side are all fun ways to work out. But don't be fooled – it's a tough workout when done with oomph and pizzazz! You'll feel re-energised, full of vitality and ready to face the day ahead (or even a good night's sleep!). I taught aquatic exercise for many years and sometimes used to jump in with my clients – such an exhilarating way to exercise!

One of the best exercises for improving lung detoxification is swimming lengths underwater – a sort of pranayama in the water. Start gently by taking one breath where you would normally have taken two – then keep building from there – greater distances in fewer breaths. Relaxation is key and in no time you'll be effortlessly swimming completely submerged.

To take the whole cleansing thing to the next level, why not get outside? Into the ocean or a lake – there's nothing like, quite literally, immersing yourself in nature to cleanse and reset your body to the natural rhythm it loves and craves.

CLEANSE CLEVER
Avoid chlorinated pools and swim in UV-light or ozone-treated pools, which are kinder to the skin, eyes and hair – not to mention lung-friendly too.

58 FULL STEAM AHEAD / STEAM

Back in the day as a child, I remember being bemused by the antics of an old uncle who had a bad cold. He sat at our kitchen table, flung a big towel over his head, leaned over a bowl of hot steaming water and took deep breaths. He immediately felt better! So why is it nowadays this old-fashioned cheap 'n' cheerful remedy that actually helped ease colds and congestion has been replaced by a multitude of expensive bad pharma cold cures that don't work?

Next time you have a cold or need to clear your sinuses, avoid the local pharmacy as there's only shelves and shelves of pills and a whole lot of advertising paraphernalia. Instead add a few drops of eucalyptus oil to a bowl of hot water, put a towel over your head and inhale the cleansing aroma for at least 15 minutes. Inhale deeply through the nose and exhale completely out through the mouth. This old-time remedy not only gets rid of the excess gunk from your lungs, nose and throat – you get a pore cleansing facial thrown in for free. Hashtag killer cleanse!

CLEANSE CLEVER
Use the cleanest water you can find – be careful the water is not scalding hot as this can hurt your nostrils!

....

59 **HERB HEAVEN** / ROSEMARY

A popular culinary herb in the Mediterranean, rosemary has a strong and energising aroma. Inhaling a few drops of rosemary essential oil on a tissue will relieve headaches, lower stress and improve mood. As an inhalant, its antiseptic properties ease sore throats, colds and flu, clearing the nasal passages and enhancing easy, comfortable breathing. When inhaled, as a bonus, it also clears the memory pathways and improves cognitive function.

Adding a few drops to your warm bath will soothe aching muscles and improve circulation, and massaging the oil into the skin using a carrier oil such as avocado or jojoba helps detoxify the liver and kidneys.

Massaging it into the scalp prevents premature hair loss and greying leaving the hair feeling and looking thicker with more shine and bounce.

CLEANSE CLEVER

Rosemary is a potent herb so must be used with awareness and safety. Always check with a qualified practitioner before you use any essential oil as some are not suitable for those with liver or kidney disease or pregnant or breast-feeding women.

....

60 **TEA-TIME** / HONEYSUCKLE TEA

I f you're suffering from a cold, a sore throat or high temperature, forget English breakfast tea and brew a cup of honeysuckle cha instead. Used in Traditional Chinese Medicine (TCM) for thousands of years, honeysuckle has tremendous medicinal kudos and drinking tea made from the pretty orange flowers of this plant (with a teaspoon of organic honey) will help alleviate the symptoms of congestion, hay fever and asthma, as well as giving a big old boost to your immune system.

Adding a few drops of honeysuckle oil to your bath will leave your skin feeling silky, and inhaling the aroma whilst relaxing in the bath will lift your mood – be prepared (and excited) though – honeysuckle can also cause an erotic dream or two!

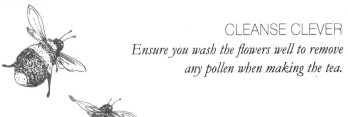

CLEANSE CLEVER

Ensure you wash the flowers well to remove any pollen when making the tea.

61 **BE A GREEN GODDESS** / ECO-FRIENDLY

Let's go eco! We all desire a clean and sparkling, sweet-smelling home and the supermarket shelves have long aisles dedicated to the latest most powerful master-blasters to ensure our kitchen, bathroom, floors, windows, ovens and tiles are squeaky clean. These chemical cleaning products and sprays emit dangerous and damaging fumes that we inhale filling our lungs with toxins, making our eyes water and irritating our skin. They can also affect our hormones and even lead to infertility.

Become a green goddess (or god) – eco-friendly and economical – and make the switch to safer and environmentally friendly green products. Bicarbonate of soda, apple cider vinegar (ACV) and lemons are just a few of the old-fashioned and perfectly adequate ways to clean around the house, wash the clothes and dishes, wipe the kitchen surfaces and ensure toilets are fresh and spotless.

As examples, bicarbonate of soda is first-rate for cleaning silver and eliminating odours in the fridge. ACV is a fabulously cheap way to make mirrors and glass shine and sparkle. And rubbing half a lemon over kitchen surfaces removes stains, leaving the kitchen smelling naturally fresh.

When disposing of old chemical products, paints, detergents and oils, take them to your local household waste site rather than pouring them down the sink and toilet. Household items such as nappies, feminine products, syringes, wet wipes and razors need to be bagged up and binned, and allow domestic fats to cool and harden before disposing in the food bin.

Check the plumbing around your house – even new-builds – to ensure gutters and gullies are correctly fitted. Pollution in our water is often due to bad house plumbing so that dirty water from dishwashers, washing machines and toilets actually goes straight into our ponds, lakes and rivers! Ask your local water company or registered plumber to fix any misconnections immediately.

The dynamic duo of baking soda and lemon juice knock the socks off any toxic store-bought stainless steel cleaner.

....

62 **CLEAR THE AIR** / AIR QUALITY

No matter how clean we keep our homes, the air inside our houses contain traces of harmful pollutants. Emissions from detergents, personal hygiene products, adhesives, carpets, upholstery, paint and plastics are just a few of the things we breathe in on a daily basis.

To improve the air quality in a green and natural way and as a bonus brighten and beautify each room is to buy air-purifying plants to freshen the air. The bedroom is a smart place to have an air freshening plant as is any room with lots of technical and computer equipment in. The kitchen is also fine place as there are often lots of electrical equipment in there too as well as fumes and smells emitted from food packaging, cleaning fluids and laundry detergents.

All plants absorb carbon dioxide and release oxygen through their leaves and help filter out the harmful toxins in the air – some have got red-carpet status, however, when it comes to air detoxification.

Here's my VIP list of air purifiers:

- Peace Lily
- Mother-in-law's Tongue (Variegated Snake Plant)
- Devil's Ivy (Money Plant)
- Gerber Daisy
- Chrysanthemum
- Aloe
- Swiss Cheese plant

CLEANSE CLEVER
When buying air-purifying plants, the bigger leaves the better. In this case size does matter!

. . . .

63 **BREATH OF FRESH AIR** / AIR CONDITIONING

The jury is still out as to whether air conditioning (AC) is bad for you or not – I suggest if you can go without it, your constitution will be better and certainly the health of your electricity bills!

Air conditioning filters need to be regularly cleaned and serviced otherwise mould and other micro-organisms grow rapidly and can cause sore throats, colds, headaches and even more serious diseases like Legionnaires' Disease.

As I live in the UK, most houses need heating rather than cooling so it's pretty easy for me to say resist switching on the AC and open the windows instead! Natural ventilation to create a breeze and blow the germs away is a much smarter route to staying cool. However if this isn't feasible, the use of ceiling fans and desk fans will help. Also drawing the curtains and keeping the blinds closed keeps the house cool, so remember to do this before you go out.

CLEANSE CLEVER
Drinking lots of water and cold water therapy will also keep you fresh.

64 **FLOAT ON AIR** / BUTEYKO METHOD

When we are stressed and anxious, our breathing tends to increase and we breathe from the upper chest so it becomes shallow and fast. In fact over-breathing is very common and so is breathing out of an open mouth (as opposed to nose breathing).

Notice if you sigh throughout the day – a possible sign of lethargy or feeling de-motivated and uninspired. I remember years ago when I worked in a job where I was subconsciously fed up, I used to sit at my desk often sighing and it wasn't until a wise work friend pointed this out, it spurred me to move on.

When you inhale and exhale through the mouth you actually lose too much carbon dioxide, and although we need to expel CO_2, too much leaves you feeling light-headed as the blood vessels constrict causing a reduced blood flow to the heart. Snoring is also a sign of incorrect breathing.

The Buteyko Method of breathing is named after a Russian doctor who developed a way to reduce his high blood pressure at just 26 years old. Correct breathing not only provides better oxygenation for our organs including our brain but improves our everyday wellbeing and enhances sound sleep. By bringing breathing to normal volume, the powerful effects of his method improves health, fitness levels, focus and mood. When breathing correctly, with mouth closed so the inhale and exhale is through the nostrils, there should hardly be any sound and it is effortless, steady and light – from the diaphragm.

As someone who exercises a lot, by practising the Buteyko Method when resting, my breathing has improved whilst doing high-intensity exercise (HIIT). One of the exercises to help you relax or if you're feeling anxious, is to place one hand on your chest and the other just above the naval and focus on the breath – notice what is going on – it may be fast and heavy or irregular. Then slow down your breathing to a gentle steady rhythm without resistance so it becomes tranquil and healing, bringing your body into the parasympathetic nervous system so you feel more relaxed.

CLEANSE CLEVER

A brisk walk is the prime time to practise nose breathing – it takes a little practice so don't be put off if you find it a challenge at first. Hashtag relax!

....

65 **HEAVEN SCENT** / REED DIFFUSER

Whenever I visit a place that has been chemically freshened, I immediately feel the harsh, poisonous fumes down the back of my throat and those commercial plug-ins, battery-operated air fresheners or carpet powder fresheners can be irritating to the eyes, skin and nose of lots of people – not to mention the damage we are doing to the environment!

So next time at the supermarket, avoid the aisle full of chemical smellies and switch to an organic essential oil reed diffuser instead – a small bunch of rattan reeds gently tied together in a glass jar that's filled with aromatherapy oils. The oil slowly climbs the sticks to bring a heavenly aroma to balance the energy in your house or place of work.

Shop-bought diffusers are usually expensive as you are paying for attractive ribbons and packaging and although they are one of my favourite gifts (to give and receive), making your own is cheaper and just as good.

The glass container or small vase ideally needs to have a small opening at the top so the aroma doesn't escape too fast or you can always use a jar with a cork lid with a hole for the reeds to pop out of. Fill the jar with a light base oil such as almond oil and a few drops of your favourite essential oil. Bunch and tie about ten little reed sticks together and place in the jar. A tip I was given by a friend was to add a small amount of alcohol (vodka is suitable – and I think she used to drink the rest!) as this enables the oil to climb up more smoothly. About once a week, turn the sticks the other way around to get a fresher stronger boost of heaven scent.

CLEANSE CLEVER

Essential oils such as lemon, grapefruit and juniper have especially cleansing properties and the aromas are just stunning too.

66 IT'S ONLY NATURAL / NATURAL FIBRES

There are many advantages to having an attractive shiny wood floor or Mediterranean-style luxurious marble tiles over wall-to-wall carpeting. In the UK, under floor heating is becoming more commonplace so more homes now are carpet-free. Carpet attracts dust and dust mites and can cause allergies and asthma, nasal congestion and irritation to the eyes and skin. And it's certainly not as easy to daily-clean a carpet after visitors have walked over it with outdoor shoes bringing in all sorts of germs. In fact whether you have carpet or natural flooring, do as they do in the East and ask everyone to leave their outdoor shoes outside!

Think about the type of soft furnishings you use around the house and aim to use natural eco-friendly fabrics for sofas, bedding, drapes and cushions. Organic cotton is soft and breathable and is grown without harmful pesticides. Non-violent silk is silk spun from open-ended cocoons and merino wool is itch-free and soft. Another natural fabric is linen, made from the fibres of our reliable friend the flax plant, and it is strong and can easily be naturally dyed.

....

67 **EAST IS EAST** / CUPPING

You may remember the paparazzi pictures of Gwyneth Paltrow and Jennifer Aniston (on separate occasions) with circular marks on their backs? They did look rather weird and shocking especially if you didn't know the marks were in fact the result of a cupping massage.

An ancient Chinese massage, cupping is now very popular and found in lots of spas and health clubs. The therapist uses small glass-like jars to create a vacuum seal usually with heat so they stick or rather suction to the body like superglue. The vacuum sucks up the skin to ease stagnation so fresh blood flows to the muscles and opens the meridians of the body to improve energy pathways. Breast pumps today stem from this idea!

Cupping is an excellent massage with many lasting and cumulative gains and is particularly suitable to ease colds, coughs and flu. It also has amazing results in fighting lung infections and lung disease, as the respiratory and blood circulations are improved and nourished by the suctioning, toxins are more easily eliminated, leaving you feeling relaxed and more able to freely breathe.

68 **NOT OUT** / EUCALYPTUS

When I was young, I remember my brother insisting his new cricket bat be made out of eucalyptus willow. As I had no idea about cricket (and still don't), I in turn bought my son a eucalyptus bat as all I knew they were strong, light and didn't split or splinter (and bound to turn my son in to a brilliant cricketer!).

I now know there are wealth of blessings to be had from eucalyptus. Native to Australia, the eucalyptus tree, apart from the cricket connection and being part of the daily diet of the Koala bear, its oil supports healthy respiration and can clear the airways easing colds, coughs and nasal congestion.

Diffusing the oil so it can be inhaled will reduce inflammation so the lungs are clear and open and rubbing a drop or two over the chest and back and also on the reflex points of the feet are tried and tested ways to relieve asthma that still works today.

Making an essential oil reed diffuser (p. 101) with eucalyptus oil is also an awesome way of keeping your home or office clear of harmful germs.

CLEANSE CLEVER
*Eucalyptus oil is antiviral and antibacterial, making it
a splendid ingredient for your eco-friendly supplies.*

....

69 **NOSE IN THE AIR** / NETI POT

Nasal irrigation has been around for centuries, and basically it's a good old-fashioned clean out of the nasal passages with a saline solution. Washing out these pathways of dust, pollen and germs has shown to give relief to sinus problems, ear blockages, colds, allergies and infections. It also decreases snoring and has been shown to help smokers who want to quit.

Using a neti pot – which looks like a baby teapot and is associated with yogis – can be bought from health food stores or online relatively cheaply. Fill the pot with warm distilled water mixed with half a teaspoon of Himalayan pink crystal salt. Stand over the sink (or in the shower). Tilt your head sideways to the left and place the spout carefully up the right top nostril and breathe through your mouth. The solution will start to flow out of the left nostril.

When you have used half the water, stand upright, blow your nose gently and repeat tilting the head the other way. Again, once done, blow your nose carefully without force. You can do this old yogic technique once or twice a day or whenever you feel the need.

CLEANSE CLEVER

As a safety precaution, do NOT share your neti pot with anyone and make sure it is washed in hot soapy water afterwards and air dried completely so it's free from germs.

....

70 **SEE THE LIGHT** / SALT LAMP

One of the best presents I received recently was a hand-carved Himalayan pink salt candle, which gives off a wonderful pinky-orange warm glow when lit. The candles can be bought online and are often sold at yoga and mind body festivals. Look out for the lamp version too – the centre of the salt rock is hollow and a light bulb is inserted to emit a soft, ambient and comforting hue and apart from making the room look pretty, salt lamps are an awesome and natural way to help purify stale indoor air. They also help counteract the electromagnetic waves given off by mobiles and PCs – so a double-whammy.

Imagine yourself at the beach standing at the salty water's edge, inhaling deeply and exhaling fully – how liberated, free and fresh you feel and how your breathing becomes easier. Although not exactly the same obviously, these lamps work on that same premise.

The health benefits of salty ionised air are well recognised to soothe inflammation and boost respiratory health as they release negative ions into the air, attract the positive ions of the pollutants around the house and hey presto, relieve the symptoms of hay fever, asthma and congestion.

CLEANSE CLEVER

Although you can buy expensive little bags to protect against the EMF emissions from your mobile phone – try turning the dang thing off and check your messages when you have time. Think digital detox!

71 SAVE YOUR BREATH / PRANAYAMA

The old phrase *'teaching grandma to suck eggs'* may come to mind as I bring up the idea of learning to breathe! I know it's a vital and largely a reflex action but we can influence its rhythm and depth, and this control can be a game-changer for cleansing and conditioning our lungs. How we breathe has far-reaching bodily effects way beyond our lungs such as improving our stress levels, how we think and our ability to control our weight.

The most recognised set of breathing exercises is found in the simple yogic practice of pranayama, meaning mastery of our life force, and has been around for thousands of years. In modern times however, we live in a world where our flight or fight switch is pretty much stuck in the ON position, so pranayama will help us effortlessly to flip the switch to OFF. And the splendid pay-off to the practice is that we spontaneously switch off and return to that easy rhythm in other times of the day outside of our practice time. The perks are huge – we'll live longer, our blood pressure is reduced, our pH level is superb, oxidative stress is lower so we look younger and finally toxins gladly flood out of our lungs!

Here's a simple little exercise to try for yourself. Begin in a comfortable cross-legged position on the floor or on a firm upright chair, and ensure your head, neck and chest are in a nice straight line, keeping the spine tall and upright.

1.   Close your eyes and simply notice how you're breathing for 30 seconds and count how long it takes you to inhale.
2.   Now you're going to create a different rhythm – make the inhale time and the exhale time the same length maintaining the natural pauses in between.
3.   Aim for just one second longer than your noticed breath in step one.
4.   Carry out 10-15 complete breaths at this rhythm.
5.   Finish by observing your breath for one minute as it returns to its comfortable natural rhythm.

CLEANSE CLEVER
Early morning is the best time to practise pranayama, especially outside in fresh air.

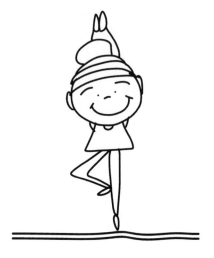

To avoid sickness eat less;
to prolong life worry less."
~ **Chu Hui Weng**

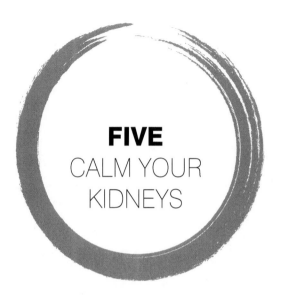

FIVE
CALM YOUR KIDNEYS

Keeping your body healthy is an expression of gratitude to the whole cosmos – the trees, the clouds, everything."
~ Thích Nhat Hanh

Our kidneys are two bean-shaped organs, each the size of a pack of cards, that cleanse and filter the blood circulating around our bodies. If there is too much water in our blood, the kidneys get rid of the extra as urine. Not enough, they then keep hold of more water. This water control system is one way our body regulates blood pressure.

The most common causes of kidney overload are large amounts of sugar in the diet, carrying extra body weight leading to high blood pressure and conventional medications causing toxic build-up. This causes a wide range of symptoms including high blood pressure, frequent urination, puffiness, tiredness, insomnia and headaches.

The following cleansing and detoxification techniques will help you establish calming kidney habits to keep you looking bright and full of vigour and able to effortlessly and naturally maintain your desired body weight.

72 **STRIKE A BALANCE** / ALKALINE ACID BALANCE

Our body fiercely strives to balance all of its unique and sensitive organs, as well as striking an overall system-wide balance – the pH level – the measure of how acidic we are – and I don't mean sharp-tongued!

In the same way that nature's acid rain kills forests and the life found in lakes and rivers, our body can't thrive in an acid state either. The pH scale is a continuum ranging between 0–14; with carbonated drinks and soda being highly acid (3); meats, fish, nuts and dairy being medium to mildly acidic (4–6); water is neutral (7); and all living edible fruits and vegetables span from 8–10 on the scale.

The foods in the 8–10 range are called alkalising or alkaline foods and interestingly enough, one of the MOST acid-tasting fruits has the most alkalising effect on the body – lemons!

It really is a piece of cake to achieve body-wide pH harmony – just follow these straightforward steps:

- Eat plenty of low-sugar **fruit and veggies**.
- **Chew your food** – saliva is alkaline too!
- **Stay hydrated**.
- **Breathe well** – oxygen alkalises your system.
- **Avoid junk food and trans fats** – enough said!
- Practise **meditation**.

- ☀ Spend some time in **natural sunlight**.

- ☀ Take some **edible clay**.

- ☀ Include more **raw food** in your diet.

CLEANSE CLEVER
Essential oils have superb alkalising effects on the body – try frankincense, myrrh or sandalwood in your massage oil or reed diffuser.

....

73 **JUST ADD WATER** / HYDRATION

We can survive without food for up to three weeks, but only three days without water. Our bodies are on average 50% water and being optimally hydrated is essential if we are to kick-ass with detoxification, bowel elimination and a strong immune system!

So how much do we need to drink each day? The *'8 x 8 rule'* is a fine place to start – that's eight 8-ounce glasses every day. Of course the cleaner your diet is, the more fruit and veggies you will be eating anyway, reducing the need for the 8 glasses – you may only need 6 or 7. Listen to your internal awareness and remember you're in charge.

In an ideal world, we would all be drinking naturally clean, pure and highly mineralised water from natural sources like wells and springs. This of course is not possible for most of us, so the next best thing is going for a glass-bottled water from a relatively local spring that will not only hydrate you but mineralise you too.

The best time to hydrate and do some power kidney flushing is first thing in the morning. I drink two glasses first thing – one, mixed with the juice from half an organic lemon to further boost cleansing – the second, plain, clean water. As well as being a top kidney cleanser, water is my number one anti-ageing remedy, regulating pH and keeping my skin looking plump and youthful at all times.

If you find it difficult or have no desire to drink your water quota, you may need more salt in your diet – try adding a pinch of Celtic sea salt (NOT table salt) to your water to boost your salt levels and also making it easier for your body to absorb the water too.

Vitamin and fruit waters may well be popular, but forget buying these at the store, as selfie versions are super-simple, easy on the pocket and way more nutritious than anything you'll find to buy. These homemade vitamin-rich waters are lifesavers for upping the amount of liquid you drink on a day-to-day basis. Try my Cucumber Cooler for yourself to hydrate, alkalise and refresh.

CUCUMBER COOLER WATER

Ingredients:

Water / 2 litres
Cucumber / ½ small – sliced
Fresh mint / 1 small bunch
Lemon juice / 1 tbsp
Sea salt / a pinch

Directions:

Combine everything in a large jug and benefit from its hydrating and cooling effects throughout the day.

CLEANSE CLEVER
Drink consistently throughout the day (small sips), even when you're not feeling thirsty as thirst is a POOR indication of hydration levels – if you feel thirsty you're ALREADY dehydrated!

74 **JUNK & DISORDERLY** / JUNK FOOD

Ditch the fast food – fast! Take a look around you – people are becoming more obese – they are in the fast lane killing themselves. But no need to panic, there's a toxic pill to remedy the damage and then there's another toxic pill to fix the side effects of the first pill! Yes we live life in the fast lane and this is an ever-expanding world, but that's certainly no excuse to rush into the supermarket filling the shopping trolley with junk – salty processed foods, fizzy drinks, sugary breakfast cereals and the wrong oils – this junk makes us extremely acidic and our kidneys just can't cope.

And as for takeaway foods – they often use the same cheap oil over and over again with added salt and sugars to make it *'tastier'* and the cheapest cuts of meat and poultry that may contain antibiotics and hormones. And it's no good throwing in a salad to counteract the negative effects – the leaves contain traces of anti-freeze to stop them wilting!

If that's not bad enough, the biggest problem with junk food is kids are being raised on it. Parents are often busy working and buying convenience foods is just that – convenient – but to the detriment of their young, growing bodies. When my kids were younger, I can't say I wasn't tempted by a packaged creamy macaroni cheese or spaghetti Bolognese after a busy day's work, but you really can't beat nutritious home-cooking.

Educate kids from an early age about healthy eating. Bring them with you to the health food store and allow them to choose the fruit and salads. Get to know your local organic butcher and make trips to the farmers' market a family event. Even my dog has ditched his pet junk food – his meals are now all organic and he devours every morsel – he just needs to learn a few more table manners and how to chew his food more slowly!

....

75 **TREAT LIKE WITH LIKE** / HOMEOPATHY

I f you are unfortunate enough to suffer kidney disorders, bladder infections or burning sensations when passing urine, the homeopathic remedy of *Cantharis Vesicatoria* can give you instant relief. Homeopathy works on the principle of taking a minute diluted dosage of a substance that if taken in large quantities would actually cause the ailment being treated! HRH Prince Charles is a fan of this complementary form of medicine.

Homeopathy originates from the Greek words – *'homeo'* meaning same and *'pathos'* meaning pain – and stems from Hippocrates' days of treating like with like. It's been in its current form for the last 200 years, developed by the German doctor, Samuel Hahnemann.

I know the jury is out on this alternative form of treatment and some say it's no more than a placebo, but I've always had excellent experiences with it – I even climbed Mt. Kilimanjaro armed with my trusted homeopathic first aid kit!

76 **LET'S TWIST AGAIN** / YOGA TWISTS

A passion of mine for many years now, yoga is an essential part of my detox toolkit. As a practice it is the ultimate holistic doctor, treating all sorts of ailments from headaches to indigestion, from muscle pain to stress. As a cleansing tonic, yogic twists are a godsend, sending rejuvenating fresh blood to the kidneys and removing any stagnation from the area as a result of the increased circulation.

Don't be put off by the complicated names for the poses – they are simply the Sanskrit names for these positions that involve a strong twist or rotation of the spine. The twist can be performed in a standing, sitting or lying position and can be held for as little as 30 seconds up to as much as 5–15 minutes, breathing deeply and evenly throughout.

Here are three of my favourites, one of each type.

STANDING – KATICHAKRASANA: Stand with your right side about 6 inches away from a wall, feet hip-distance apart. Without moving your feet and hips, place both hands on the wall at chest height to create the spinal twist. Press your right hand deeper into the wall whilst maintaining the levelness of the hips so you can rotate further. Breathe steadily, drawing your shoulder blades downwards and lifting your chest. Repeat the other way, standing with your left side to the wall and pressing the left hand into the wall to revolve.

SITTING – ARDHA MATSYENDRASANA: Sitting up tall on the floor, stretch your left leg straight out in front and hug your right knee into your chest, your heel on the floor in line with the sitting bone. Maintain the hug with your left arm and place your right-cupped hand at the base of the spine behind you. Twist to look over the right shoulder. Breathe deeply and relax into the stretch as you grow taller, twisting further. Repeat on the other side.

LYING – JATHARA PARIVARTANASANA: Lie on your back and draw your knees in towards the chest. Stretch your arms out to the sides and allow your knees to gently fall over to your right-hand side keeping both shoulders on the floor if you can. Feel your spine twist more and more with each breath. Repeat with knees going the other way.

These poses are simple and super-effective at rejuvenating your kidneys as well as all other organs in the abdomen.

CLEANSE CLEVER

Synchronise your breathing with your twist movement – use your exhale to deepen a little further into the twist.

77 PINS & NEEDLES / ACUPUNCTURE

Traditional Chinese Medicine (TCM) and specifically acupuncture has been practised in China for thousands of years, having many healing effects on the body, including relieving pain, reducing inflammation, restoring balance and stimulating detoxification.

The ultra-fine stainless steel needles used by modern acupuncturists started out as slivers of stone, bone or even gold and silver, and are placed on specific points of the body related to the area of concern, often nowhere near the problem area. The kidneys, for example, have treatment points on the inner foot!

Many people unfortunately forego treatment because of the misconception that getting pricked with needles actually hurts. The truth is you will feel something but not anything sharp and not when the needle is first inserted. I can only describe it as being like a small weight on the area. Your acupuncturist may also use words like, achy, tingly or warm and these are excellent descriptions too, but you need to experience it for yourself.

TCM practitioners highly recommend acupuncture for detoxification and believe the more toxic you are, the stronger the cleansing will be. So even if there is some discomfort involved, this *'free from negative side effects'*, is a safe and effective therapy and may be the detox game-changer you've been looking for! Also consider using a shakti mat.

CLEANSE CLEVER

Take it easy after your acupuncture treatment – skip exercise that day, take a nice hot bath and go to bed early.

....

78 **TEATOX** / STINGING NETTLE

Mostly thought of as a weed that *'fights back'*, the stinging nettle has been used for centuries as a remedy for a whole bunch of maladies, as well as in the cooking pot, which eradicates the nasty sting.

As usual Mother Nature has combined a killer set of ingredients in a plant that gets such a bum rap – it's packed with calcium, chlorophyll, magnesium, iron, chromium, zinc and vitamins A, C, D and K.

Its strong diuretic quality helps flush mineral build-up and toxins away from the kidneys, getting it on to the kidney cleanse A-list. A hot brew of nettle leaf tea is the most popular tipple but can also be used as a substitute in any dish calling for spinach – it tastes pretty similar but you get much more bang for your buck!

CLEANSE CLEVER

Nettle tea can interact with some traditional medications – consult with your medical practitioner before use.

79 **PURE PRIMAL** / PALEO DIET

Endorsed by Matthew McConaughey, Megan Fox, Jessica Biel and Miley Cyrus, the Paleo or caveman diet is gathering huge momentum in the health world, topping the Google diet search list in recent times. But what is it exactly and can it help us with our detoxification efforts?

The eating plan is based on the idea that eating like our ancestors in the Palaeolithic era (more than 10,000 years ago) is more suited to our biology than our modern-day diet. Here's the no-go list of foods: no refined, processed foods (savoury and sweet); no sweet fruits or juices; no grains, bread or GMO foods; no seed oils; and no dairy. And the yes list: vegetables, tart fruits, nuts, meat, eggs, coconut oil, grass-fed butter and olive oil.

At first glance this seems too restrictive for day-to-day living, but if we reconsider with our cleanse-tinted specs on, it ticks a LOT of low-toxin boxes – getting rid of sugar, dairy, processed food and grains will have a GIANT impact on detoxing our body. The trick is balancing the macronutrients (carbs, fats and proteins) of the remaining foods. The ratio can be adjusted according to individual needs but the bulk of the diet should consist of energy-rich fats – lots of good fats that our bodies love to use as their primary fuel.

The biggest challenge of the Paleo paradigm is avoiding the trap of eating large amounts of protein, causing high levels of uric acid in our blood and overtaxing the kidneys as they struggle to get rid of it. Paleo is NOT a high-protein diet and can be a superb elimination diet to get a head start on weight loss, leading to a youthful, healthier lifestyle.

CLEANSE CLEVER

Simple, clean eating doesn't have to be boring – remember your friends: garlic, ginger, cayenne, mint and lemon.

80 **ON THE GO** / DIURETICS

Proper hydration is essential to help flush the kidneys of harmful toxins and is even more important when we add diuretics into the mix. These substances found in food and herbs to increase the rate of urination, helping to excrete toxins from the kidneys, lowering blood pressure and dropping extra water weight. Most high-water-content fruits and vegetables have diuretic properties and here are some of the heavy-hitters for flushing those kidneys – cranberries, watermelon, lemon, cucumber, beets, carrots, celery and cabbage.

Even more powerful kidney tonics are the super-heavyweight herbs of the diuretic world – parsley, ginger, dandelion leaf, stinging nettle, garlic, fennel, horseradish and its Japanese cousin; wasabi.

Of course Mother Nature is a fabulous multi-tasker, so being a diuretic is often just one of many hats that these food can wear. Others include – high in antioxidants, cancer fighting, heart protective and cholesterol balancing.

One of my favourite kidney-kind elixirs is so simple and is just four ingredients to cleanse internally and as a beauty bonus, reflected in a glowing, younger-looking complexion!

FRESH FLUSH JUICE

Ingredients

Carrots / 2 medium
Cucumber / 1 medium
Raw Beet / ½ medium
Raw Ginger / ½ inch chunk or to taste

Directions:

Push all ingredients through the juicer starting with the ginger and prepare to flush!

....

81 **SALT OF THE EARTH** / SEA SALT

Salt has been part of our lives for countless millennia. It's been a valuable trade commodity, it's featured in many religious ceremonies and it's even been used as currency. It's where the word salary comes from!

Whilst we cannot live without salt, the white stuff we call table salt (sodium chloride) is a far cry from a whole and healthy natural salt, having been heat treated, stripped of over 84 essential minerals and has had nasty chemicals added to stop caking, etc. A form of aluminium is one of these additives and is a potential cause of Alzheimer's disease. Table salt of course is an easy target and simple to address. Exchange it for top-quality sea salt like Atlantic grey salt.

Beware, harmful sodium chloride lurks in the most unexpected places – breakfast cereals, pasta sauces, veggie burgers, ketchup, cheese slices, canned veggies, low fat labels, salad dressings, pre-cooked rice, and so. Eliminating processed foods due to their high-salt value is just one reason to banish them from the shopping list. Our kidneys will breathe a sigh of relief as they pack their bags and go – leaving us feeling revived, less bloated and less thirsty!

82 **THE SPICE OF LIFE** / GINGER

fell in love with the tangy, fresh and zesty ginger many moons ago and now use it on a near-daily basis. I cook with it, drink it in juices and teas, bathe my feet in it, massage my body with it and add it to body scrubs. Mother Nature certainly broke the mould with this insanely beneficial root used in many south Asian cultures of the long distant past and still popular today.

This ugly-ducking root certainly has loads of health advantages – it's anti-inflammatory, helps with motion-sickness and lowers blood pressure. It's a natural pain-killer, easing cold and flu symptoms and helps maintain normal blood circulation. It is also unrivalled in easing indigestion or tummy upsets and lastly offers protection to the kidneys in the form of powerful antioxidants.

I tend to use ginger as it comes from nature, in root form, but if that's not available, a high-quality organic powder can be substituted although it is a little spicier in flavour!

Here's my detox bath recipe – you'll love it I'm sure.

BATH BLISS DETOX

Ingredients:

Epsom salts / ½ cup
Fresh ginger / ½ cup freshly juiced
Essential oil / A few drops of your fave aroma

Directions:

After running your bath add the bath bliss ingredients. Get in and soak for 15–20 minutes. Emerge feeling recharged, relaxed and youthful.

....

83 **CATCH OF THE DAY** / OILY FISH

Unless you've been on a serious digital detox and haven't seen the news, you'll be well aware we all need oily fish in our diets. But what exactly are the purifying perks and how often do we need to eat it to gain the health benefits?

The perks come from the high levels of omega-3 fats – a particular polyunsaturated fat that helps lubricate the joints, decrease inflammation, fight wrinkles, protect vision, protect the heart, banish brain fog, clear cholesterol and protect the kidneys. That's quite a list!

The highest sources of this superfood in the aquatic world come from FRESH cold-water fish like wild-caught salmon, sardines, herring and mackerel. At least two servings a week of your chosen oily fish is suggested. And for those who like Japanese food, a dish of sashimi (raw fish) is my favourite omega-3 rich meal, complete as nature intended – just add a dash of spicy wasabi condiment for its diuretic properties and your kidneys will be in detox heaven!

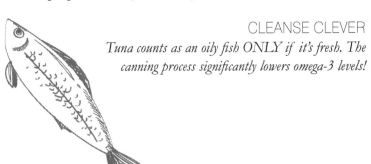

84 **KALE & HEARTY** / KALE

Those of you who already love your daily green smoothie will probably be using kale as one of your go-to green ingredients – not surprising really, since it's delicious, nutritious, antioxidant-packed and has anti-inflammatory strengths.

But did you know that consuming excessive raw kale may be increasing your risk of kidney stones? Kale has a dark side in the form of a so-called anti-nutrient called oxalic acid – the plant's natural self-defence against being eaten by animals and insects. In our digestive tract however, it limits absorption of some nutrients, especially calcium and iron, by latching onto them and creating oxalate crystals. It's these crystals that can contribute to kidney stones! Strategies to combat the anti-nutrient, however, are quite simple to put in place.

Firstly, even though cooking does not destroy oxalic acid, it releases one third of the toxin into the cooking water, which should be discarded. And secondly, just being mindful of the potential risk and NOT eating huge amounts of raw kale in one sitting will help greatly. The bad bugs in our gut absolutely love oxalic acid so make sure your detox army of friendly bacteria are fully trained and present.

CLEANSE CLEVER
Eat calcium-rich raw dairy with your high oxalic acid foods to balance their calcium-robbing tendencies!

....

85 **WAKE UP & SMELL THE COFFEE** / CAFFEINE

We love it and drink tons of the stuff and it's THE most valuable legally traded food commodity in the world. Discovered in Ethiopia, coffee is now grown in Asia, Central and South America, the Caribbean and Pacific islands, as well as its native Africa. It's now a daily ritual for millions all over the globe, but what's it doing to our health?

Like all foods, if taken in excess, coffee too has a shadowy side that includes disrupting sleep, elevating blood pressure, staining teeth and hampering absorption of some minerals and vitamins. However, Mother Nature always strives for balance and with this little bean she has helped reduce the risk of asthma, Alzheimer's Disease, diabetes, Parkinson's Disease, heart problems, depression and kidney stones.

In summing up, although I eliminated coffee from my diet years ago as I couldn't ever stick at one cup, this complicated little bean can be a superfood when treated more like a medicinal herb to be used sparingly rather than a fix or multiple-times-a-day energy drink. Keep chanting the *'less is more'* mantra and buy the best organic coffee you can afford. Coffee's mild diuretic effect and feel-good vibe will keep your kidneys flushing and your outlook sunny!

CLEANSE CLEVER

Try bumping up the good fat content of your coffee by adding raw grass-fed milk or grass-fed butter a.k.a. 'Bulletproof Coffee', this extends the feel-good vibe for longer and boosts brainpower!

86 THE BERRY THING / CRANBERRIES

Cranberries probably give you more bang for your buck for kidney cleansing than any other food, but did you know it's one of only a trio of major fruits native to the US? Blueberries and concord grapes are the other two.

The crimson, pea-sized and acid-tasting cranberry is packed with detox rewards, including strong antioxidants to combat urinary tract

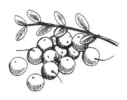

infections (UTIs), natural antibacterial action for oral hygiene and to combat plaque, and helps tip the balance in favour of the good bacteria in the gut by flushing out candida and other excess fungi from our system.

So as *'a dog is for life not just for Christmas'*, so too are these versatile little red gems – consider including them throughout the year to boost detox, anti-ageing and weight-loss routines. Below is my flu-fighting and detox panacea for year-round use!

CRANBERRY CLEANSER

Ingredients:

Mango / ½ small
Cranberries / ¼ cup
Pomegranate / ½ – seeds only
Ginger / ½ inch chunk or to taste
Turmeric / ½ inch chunk or ½ tsp turmeric powder
Lemon / 1 – juiced

Directions:

Pop the lot in a blender with enough water to cover and whiz until smooth. Add more water for a lighter blend. Drink and cleanse to your kidneys' content!

CLEANSE CLEVER

When cranberries are mixed with copious amounts of sugar you can say bye-bye to their health blessings! Replace sugar with stevia in your homemade cranberry sauce.

87 **SQUEAKY CLEAN** / MUCUS

You may not immediately think of food as being the cause of mucus build-up in the lungs and nose, but if you consider dairy, salt, sugar, nicotine and trans fats to be your buddies, you may need to have a little rethink.

Your body is like a dance club with mucus as the bouncer, keeping out the riff-raff. You'll see how effective it is at managing undesirable dust when you blow your nose after spending time in a very dusty room or on the London tube – lots of little dots of dust trapped in mucus like flies on fly-paper!

Excess mucus however, is a perfect example of your detox system being revved up to cleanse your body of toxins. So if you feel constantly bunged up then consider unfriending dairy, salt, sugar, nicotine and trans fats, and friending the following instead: garlic (p. 77), steam (p. 94), water (p. 111) and deep breathing (p. 106).

Try my Breathe-Easy remedy to help keep you clear and open.

BREATHE-EASY JUICE SHOT

Ingredients:

Pear / 2 organic
Raw ginger / ½ inch chunk or to taste
Raw honey / ½ tsp

Directions:

Juice the ginger and pears, then blend in the honey – knock it back and take a deep breath!

CLEANSE CLEVER

Friendly bugs not only line our intestines but also our lungs – consuming probiotic foods helps reduce mucus build-up in the lungs too.

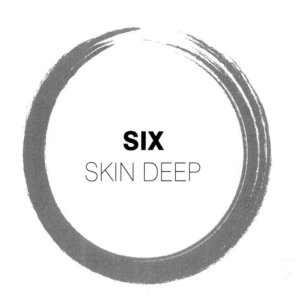

SIX
SKIN DEEP

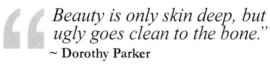

Beauty is only skin deep, but ugly goes clean to the bone."
~ **Dorothy Parker**

Our skin is our first line of protection from our day-to-day toxin-laden environment and this even includes our clothes if not chosen mindfully. It also allows us to expel tiny amounts of toxins in the water we excrete to regulate body temperature. More importantly and often overlooked, our skin is super-effective in absorbing whatever it comes in contact with, be that creams and lotions, fabrics and furnishings or even chemicals in the water we bathe in.

Obviously like our kitchen sieve, when not cared for or cleaned properly, it gets clogged and starts to develop a life of its own! In skin terms this could show up as skin infections, dryness, rashes or breakouts.

I believe the secret to gorgeous, radiant skin is a blend of science, common sense, lifestyle choices and a simple daily skincare routine.

....

88 **UNDER THE SUN** / SUNSHINE

As with all things in life, moderation is the key, and sun exposure is no exception. Studies have shown that the *'sunshine vitamin'*, vitamin D actually prevents many types of cancer, which is ironic really considering 90% of skin cancer is actually related to damage caused by too much sun worshiping. Too much sun means more wrinkles, collagen breakdown and skin pigmentation.

The sun can be our best friend, we just need to be sensible and safe, avoiding 10am–4pm and always dress to impress – natural non-toxic sunscreen (SPF 15 or higher) when fully exposed, otherwise wide-brimmed hats, sunglasses, long sleeved tops and trousers.

As well as topping up our vitamin D levels, our new BFF comes with other detox delights – more vitamin D equals happy, healthy liver and kidney function as well as regular digestion and a better mood. Keep chanting my mantra *'less is more'* and your sunny relationship will stand the test of time!

CLEANSE CLEVER

Avoid slapping on too much sunscreen – more
doesn't mean safer. Balance is the key.

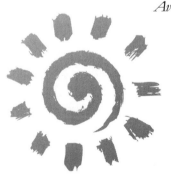

89 **SAVE YOUR OWN SKIN** / MOISTURISE

Nourishing our bodies doesn't start and stop at filling our stomach – the skin needs nurturing *'food'* too. Unfortunately the skin can be compared to an unsupervised toddler in the kitchen, consuming everything and anything it can get its hands on. The protective outer layer absorbs about 60% of whatever we feed it so that's still a lot of clearing up for the liver to deal with when the harmful chemicals arrive.

The good news is, however, non-toxic skincare ranges are becoming more available and affordable, so check your existing product range for all-natural options, and ditch them if they contain junk.

Read the small print though, as the all-natural and organic slogans can just be marketing camouflage for the unsuspecting buyer and may not be all they first appeared to be.

CLEANSE CLEVER
*The shorter the list of ingredients your moisturiser
has the better, assuming you've brought your
electron microscope with you to read it!*

....

90 **SMELL A RAT** / BODY ODOUR

We all gag when we catch a whiff of someone's B.O! And although sweating of course is as natural and necessary as breathing, bad and stale body odour is optional. If you reach for a roll-on, stick or spray to neutralise the scent – think again!

These chemical deodorants often contain lots of horrible properties the body won't thank you for such parabens, PEGs, hormone-disrupting fragrances, antibacterials, petrochemicals and aluminium compounds. The latter is being linked with breast cancer and widely used in deodorants as well as other beauty products.

Many more holistic choices are now available and my advice is to try a few out for yourself. Remember our skin chemistry is as individual as our fingerprints, so whatever a friend recommends as working like a charm may not necessary suit you.

CLEANSE CLEVER

Spritzing with apple cider vinegar, then wiping dry, can help to eliminate those unattractive underarm odours.

....

91 **HOLY COW!** / DAIRY

Due to our overly sweet Western diets, the sugar in milk (lactose) has become the final straw to break the camel's back (or rather the cow's back?) To add insult to injury, our milk has also become so de-natured through pasteurisation that to our digestive tract it is considered hazardous rather than healing.

We are all wonderfully unique though, and some of us are able to tolerate milk and dairy products more than others – up to about 30% of the population however, is estimated to be lactose intolerant. If you have ongoing skin breakouts and rashes, you may have to consider ditching dairy for a week or two and re-evaluate your skin and overall vitality afterwards.

The gains may surprise you. Many of my clients are amazed at how rejuvenating being non-dairy can be. Depending on your tolerance level you may be able to graze occasionally and if you're lucky enough to find raw unpasteurised dairy products at your local farmers' market

– go for that, otherwise your best bet is plain, unsweetened yoghurt containing lots of probiotics.

CLEANSE CLEVER

Revered in Ayurveda as a medicine, ghee is a fantastic way to keep butter in your diet – it's still butter fat, but minus all traces of lactose – a.k.a. clarified butter.

....

92 **RUB UP THE RIGHT WAY** / MASSAGE

In my mind, massage is THE ultimate skin and immune system tonics. The pressure and movements of an experienced therapist's hands act like a skin workout, stimulating and boosting the body's natural detox and lymphatic system.

There are many flavours to choose from including Swedish, Ayurvedic, Thai yoga, shiatsu, hot stone, aromatherapy, acupressure and reflexology. Some are performed fully-clothed, like Thai Yoga massage, and others, Ayurvedic or Swedish massage for example, the therapist kneads and rubs nourishing oils directly into the skin to trigger a deeper cleansing action.

Finding a therapist who is a good fit to your personality and needs can be a little tricky at first, so recommendations from friends are my favourite way of discovering one. Also health clubs and beauty spas can be an excellent option too.

CLEANSE CLEVER

Arrive for your massage on an empty stomach and drink plenty of fluids afterwards to keep hydrated and flush those toxins.

93 **SCRUB & BRUSH** / EXFOLIATE

Our skin is constantly regenerating itself and on average we shed 50,000 cells every minute – about half a kilo of dead skin cells every year! As one of our primary elimination exits, it's essential to keep it clear of any build-up so toxins can freely leave. Exfoliation is the quick and simple answer, and an invigorating way to slough off the dead cells is to use a dry body brush, a loofah or a mesh puff so you gently tingle and feel velvety all over.

Sea salt body scrubs are a favourite of mine and my Lemon Pie Scrub below is a fabulous homemade exfoliator that leaves you feeling squeaky clean and energised.

And a free way to get a lasting tan after drenching yourself in vitamin D on the beach? Just use some fine sand grains and give yourself a quick invigorating scrub. Not only do you lose the excess dry cells, it's a natural way to stop unsightly and annoying peeling! When in Rio recently, the fine golden grains of Ipanema beach were just sublime!

LEMON PIE BODY SCRUB

Ingredients:

White sugar / 1 cup
Coconut oil / ½ cup
Lemon essential oil / 20 drops

Directions:

Combine all the ingredients in a large bowl – then divide into glass storage pots. Easy-peasy lemon pie scrub!

CLEANSE CLEVER

Bear in mind, the skin on the face is way more sensitive than the rest of your body so use specifically designed facial products and moisturise, moisturise, moisturise after any scrub – face and body!

94 **SWEAT IT OUT!** / HIIT

M y career in the health and fitness industry started with a passion for Jane Fonda, legwarmers and aerobics classes and although we've moved on from then, the *'sweat it out'* mantra is still going strong.

Things have changed since those days though in terms of intensity and the time recommended. Gone are the one hour hi or lo-impact classes on studio timetables and these days it's all about HIIT – that's High Intensity Interval Training to the uninitiated – all-out maximum effort for say twenty seconds followed by a short rest of ten seconds, then rinse and repeat for as little as four minutes.

Tabata is one variety of this workout and it certainly ticks all the boxes when it comes to body cleansing – massage for the lymphatic system, sweating for the skin, a great lung detox and helping us also to maintain a healthy body weight and lessening the strain on the liver.

CLEANSE CLEVER
If you've been pretty inactive for a long period of time, check with a medical professional before your first HIIT session.

....

95 **HOT DAMN!** / DYNAMIC YOGA

I 've been in love with yoga since my very first downward dog years ago, and whilst there are many styles to choose from, the dynamic, energetic styles of Bikram, Ashtanga and the like are close to my heart. So rejuvenating and cleansing!

Hot yoga or Bikram Yoga has been around since the 70s but only really reached boiling point in popularity in the past 10–15 years, with celebs like David Beckham, George Clooney and Jennifer Aniston turning the heat up. Traditionally lasting 90 minutes, the class is made up of a set sequence of 26 postures, performed in the same order each time – the big difference to conventional yoga classes is the high temperature of the studio – 105°F (40.6°C) and 40% humidity. For all heat lovers, me included, it's a real plus to practice yoga in such a high temperature – your muscles literally melt into positions that would otherwise take a lot more coaxing.

Ashtanga yoga has quite a similar format to a Bikram class – a sequence of moves called the *'primary series'* being performed in each class – there's no added heat though, but the constant flowing movement combined with powerful, deep breathing generate such internal heat that the need for any external heat will be far from your thoughts.

The skin detox perks of these yoga styles are sizzling – and even though yoga already has a strong cleansing element, the heating aspect catapults elimination and purging skyward, leaving your skin glowing and radiant. Check online listings for a nearby class to enjoy this natural movement method of detoxification.

CLEANSE CLEVER

If you feel dizzy or light-headed during class, sit down and take a few sips of water. Listen to your body!

....

96 **SMOOTH SAILING** / GREEN SMOOTHIE

Vibrant, healthy skin can be just a nutritious and delicious smoothie away – a green smoothie to be precise. I know it may not sound particularly appealing after glancing at the ingredient list – spinach AND pineapple in the same glass – but it is quite delicious, and only needs just a little bit of practice to get the Goldilocks taste that's completely right for you.

The basic recipe is 50% fruit, 40% leafy greens and 10% good fats (avocado, coconut oil or nuts) – simply pop everything into a blender and within seconds you'll be at Cleanse Central travelling to bright youthful skin continuing all the way along the road to longevity.

SKIN SUPPORT SMOOTHIE

Ingredients:

Green leaves / 1 cup of your choice – spinach, kale, salad greens
Nut milk or coconut water / 1 cup
Water / 1 cup
Pineapple / 1 cup (peeled)
Avocado / 1 small

Directions:

Blend the lot in a high-speed blender until smooth and enjoy.

CLEANSE CLEVER
If you're a newbie to green smoothies, start with the mild leafy greens like spinach – then little by little add some kale until you're up to a 50/50 mix.

97 **COLD COMFORT** / COLD WATER THERAPY

Our modern showers and baths obviously haven't been around for as long as we humans have been on the planet, but crystal-clear mountain lakes, cascading waterfalls and thirst-quenching rivers have. Many ancient civilizations, including my Greek ancestors and the Japanese, believed immersion in cold water to be the ultimate cleansing for health and spirit.

In modern times our showers give us access to an easy skin-cleansing treat. After you have finished the *'wash-cycle'* move on to the *'cleanse-cycle'* by turning the temperature up to as hot as you can bear for 30 seconds and then alternate with the lowest cold setting for 30 seconds. Do this three to four times and you'll step out feeling aglow and flushed – in the best possible way!

Here's another wildly beneficial and rejuvenating, low-temperature therapy that's super-simple to do at home – partially fill a bath with cold water to about ankle depth and go for a little paddle – use ice if you're in hotter climes to really sink that temperature. I know it sounds a little pedestrian (excuse the pun) to have much of a cleansing effect but believe me your circulation and metabolism will leap up a few gears in reaction to the icy temperatures!

CLEANSE CLEVER
Contrary to popular belief studies have proven cold showers actually raise libido and testosterone levels in men – building energy and strength.

....

98 **TRIP THE LIGHT FANTASTIC** / INFRARED SAUNA

As well as providing vitamin D, there's also the feel-good factor when exposing our body to sunlight and even the heat and light from the winter sun can feel incredibly rejuvenating. Infrared saunas tap into this by using the non-harmful part of the sun's radiation (infrared waves) to produce a wonderful alternative to the traditional sauna experience. Gone is the overwhelming instant heat, replaced by a gentle heating from within.

Researches and doctors in China discovered the healing power of infrared waves about 20 years ago, leading to the emergence of infrared technology including infrared saunas. Heat therapy with traditional saunas, however, is well documented for its terrific cleansing and detoxification effects. Any time our blood circulation is upped, our detox system also gets cranked up too, recognising the faster metabolism as the ultimate time to declutter any toxins in storage. A study by the British Medical Association proved that those who take saunas regularly (2–3 per week) reduce their incidence of colds and flu by over 65%.

CLEANSE CLEVER

For best detoxification results, wait at least one to two hours after eating before taking a sauna.

99 **A DOSE OF SALTS** / EPSOM SALTS

Epsom salts (magnesium sulphate) takes its name from the quaint spa town, Epsom in the UK, and they became recognised for their medicinal properties back in the late 1600s. Using salts to heal various ailments and promote detoxification, however, has been around for much longer. The ancient Greeks and Chinese physicians knew all too well the godsends of immersing their patients in salty water. We've all heard of people flocking to The Dead Sea in Israel to heal illnesses and skin complaints for the same reason, and now we can quite simply recreate this effect using our own bath.

Just pop three cups of Epsom salts into warm bath water to upgrade your regular bathing experience to a first-class cleansing and anti-ageing spa ritual. You'll emerge with baby-soft skin and topped up with purifying minerals that continue their cleansing skills well after your immersion time.

....

100 **SCENT-SATIONAL** / ESSENTIAL OILS

Did you know our noses can distinguish more than 10,000 different scents and our sense of smell is our only sense that has direct paths to the part of our brain linked to memory? I'm sure before now, you've caught a whiff of an aroma and can immediately conjure a detailed back-story from just the smell as the trigger. The age-old art of aromatherapy uses the power of plant essential oils for a variety of restorative, cleansing and purging results. The complex chemical composition of the oils have a profound effect on our bodies as well as our mindset.

We glean the favour of essential oils in a mixture of ways – we can smell them via candles, reed diffusers or burners; we can inhale them in steam rooms or by a simple basin and towel set-up; we can add them to a detox bath; or we can absorb them through our skin during a soothing massage. My top three scent-sational essential oils I use for detoxing are grapefruit, juniper berry and rosemary.

101 **AT THE SHARP END** / SHAKTI MAT

Good circulation has everything to do with your skin's health and its ability to expel excess toxins. Think of a shopping centre on Saturday afternoon – lots of movement, hustle and bustle, exactly how we want the blood cells in our intricate circulation system to be – always on the move and busy *'shopping'*. Stagnation or sluggish flow anywhere in the body leads to toxins accumulating, causing chaos and overloading for the liver. A novel way to get your circulation back on point is quite literally to stimulate your skin by lying on a modern-day Indian-style bed of nails or Shakti mat.

Now I know the sex appeal for doing this is sub-zero, but have a look at the pros confirmed by Russian scientists – decreased inflammation, strengthened immune system, increased metabolism and decreased stress levels. It also alleviates depression, leaving you with a sense of wellness and calm.

Does it hurt? Well, yes and no – the initial response is your body screaming *'enough already'*, but after a little *'mind over spikes'* the pain reduces to a comfortable ache. I find once past the three to five minute mark, it's a whole lot easier. Hang in there, arrive at a *'happy place'* and allow the detoxifying, stimulating and healing effect to melt through you.

CLEANSE CLEVER
Also known as AcuMat or Spike Mat, you can hike up your bang-for-buck by lying with your legs up the wall while the mat is under your back.

FAQ

Q: I feel fine so why do I need to incorporate Daily Detox into my lifestyle?

A: As the saying goes, *'You cannot miss what you never had'*, and by all means remain *'feeling fine'*. However I firmly believe that by taking action to move your mind and body closer to a cleaner lifestyle and start experiencing the marvellous perks to your constitution and wellbeing, you'll stop *'feeling fine'* and start *'feeling fantastic'*.

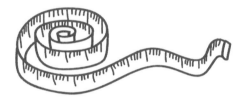

Q: Can I use Daily Detox for weight-loss?

A: Yes you can – you will notice you will lose excess weight naturally and steadily and then continuing on your clean healthy path will ensure you maintain the weight that is right for you.

Q: How do I know whether I am 'toxic' and need to up my cleansing efforts?

A: The Toxin Tally (p. 22) at the start of the book will give you an idea, and implementing my suggestions will certainly give you more va-va-voom and enhance longevity. If you are unsure or have any concerns, then always consult your doctor.

GLOSSARY

ACID REFLUX: a.k.a. heartburn, is the pain experienced when stomach acid needed to digest food escapes back into the gullet – causing a burning sensation.

ALZHEIMER'S DISEASE: a condition that gradually destroys memory and other important brain activities.

AMINO ACIDS: used in every cell of our body to build protein necessary to live.

ANAEMIA: a blood condition where there is a decrease in the number of red blood cells that carry life-giving oxygen around the body.

ARTHRITIS: painful inflammation of the joints – can be a result of trauma, infection or age.

AYURVEDA: considered by many to be the oldest healing science, Ayurveda means *'The Science of Life'*, and originated in India more than 5,000 years ago. The primary focus of Ayurvedic medicine is to promote good health, rather than fight disease and illness.

CANDIDA: one of the best-known bad bacteria (a.k.a. yeast) that live in our gut – a quality high fibre diet and healthy immune system will usually keep its numbers manageable but if left unchecked it can cause thrush, vaginal yeast infections, skin rashes and weakened immune function.

CHAKRAS: in yoga, our body's seven basic energy centres that allow *'life energy'* to flow into and out of our aura – correlate to colours, body functions, sounds and more.

CIRRHOSIS: sever damage to the liver caused by alcoholism or hepatitis.

CORTISOL: our body's best-known stress hormone – released in reaction to either physical or emotional stress.

DIABETES: a condition of having too much sugar in the blood.

ESSENTIAL FATTY ACIDS (EFA): we can make most fats we need to thrive from within our body, however, we cannot synthesise essential fatty acids – they must be obtained from food. Two of these EFAs are called omega-3 and omega-6 fatty acids.

FLAVONOID: natural substances found in all plants giving them their dazzling bright hues, e.g. quercitin.

FREE RADICALS: our bodies naturally produce free radicals as a result of internal energy processes. Stress, trans fats and toxins from pollution and poor lifestyle choices also create free radicals.

GLYCAEMIC INDEX (GI): a measure of the impact on blood sugar levels, by food containing carbohydrate. The range being 0–55 (LOW GI), 56–69 (MEDIUM GI) and 70–100 (High GI). Apples for example have a GI of 36 and Cornflakes a GI of 81.

GOUT: painful swelling and inflammation of one or more joints – most often the big toe – caused by high levels of uric acid in the blood.

HEPATITIS: inflammation of the liver caused by toxins, infections, alcohol and certain medications.

IRRITABLE BOWEL SYNDROME (IBS): a common disorder affecting the large intestine (colon) – symptoms include: cramping, abdominal pain, bloating gas, diarrhoea and constipation. These symptoms however, don't cause permanent colon damage.

KOMBUCHA: ancient Chinese fermented beverage a.k.a. *'Immortal Health Elixir'* – made with tea, sugar, bacteria and yeast.

KEFIR: originating in Russia – a tangy, fermented milk drink, similar in flavour to yoghurt.

LEAKY GUT SYNDROME: a condition where our gut lining becomes dangerously weakened – allowing food and other toxins to pass unhindered and easily in to our bloodstream.

LYMPHATIC SYSTEM: an important part of our immune system – maintains our fluid levels, filters our blood and destroys bacteria.

MUCOID PLAQUE: thick build-up on our intestinal walls of accumulated toxins from our diet – optimal healing and detoxification cannot occur in the presence of this mucoid plaque.

OFFAL: a.k.a. organ meats – the nutrient-rich organs of animals – kidneys, liver, heart, etc.

PARABENS: shorthand for chemical toxins found a never-ending list of pharmacy products including shampoos and conditioners, moisturisers, shaving products, personal lubricants, spray tans, makeup and toothpaste.

PARASYMPATHETIC NERVOUS SYSTEM: the *'relax and renew'* part of our autonomic nervous system responsible for bringing us back to balance after experiencing stress or pain.

PARKINSON'S DISEASE: a gradual condition affecting the nervous system leading to muscle tremors, stiffness and slow movement.

PEG: known skin carcinogen used in cosmetic ranges.

PINEAL GLAND: a small gland in the brain responsible for melatonin production.

SANSKRIT: one of the very old official languages of India, but no longer spoken – still used today to name yoga poses.

SYMPATHETIC NERVOUS SYSTEM: the *'fight or flight'* part of our autonomic nervous system responsible for producing an immediate response to dangerous emergency situations.

TRADITIONAL CHINESE MEDICINE (TCM): still used by millions all over the planet, the ancient healing art of TCM has been around for thousands of years – strongly focused on observing nature to create balance in our body.

URIC ACID: a natural by-product of our metabolism – elevated levels caused by high-sugar diets and certain drugs can lead to gout.

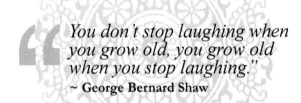

You don't stop laughing when you grow old, you grow old when you stop laughing."

~ George Bernard Shaw

★ BONUS ★
MY TOP 7 GREEN JUICE RECIPES

These seven pure, cleansing and all-natural juice recipes will move you into the detox fast lane and keep your inner purification systems on your side. Clearly organic produce is best for extra oomph, but the blessings gained of using well-scrubbed non-organic fruit and veggies FAR outweigh not juicing at all!

Each juice contains ONLY three ingredients – great foundations to start building on. Feel free to fine-tune and fiddle with the blends – these are just some of my go-to starting blends – play with them and make them yours, be creative!

GETTING STARTED

It really is quite simple – here's a few basic pointers.

Getting the right ratio of ingredients is the real magic of juicing – what I call the balancing the **THREE Bs – base, beauty and brawn**.

Meet the **BASE** *ingredients:*

Cucumber, Celery, Courgette, Spinach, Kale, Romaine – all the green earthy flavours.

Add some **BEAUTY** *to the mix:*

Apple, Watermelon, Pineapple, Berries, Papaya, Orange, Cranberry – sweet and juicy delights.

And last but not least, a bit of **BRAWN***:*

Ginger, Cayenne, Lemon, Garlic, Fennel, Watercress, Turmeric, Mint, Coriander, Parsley, Wheatgrass, Dandelion Leaf – packed with zest and punch.

You're aiming for a juice that has the following proportions: **70% BASE, 25% BEAUTY AND 5% BRAWN**, but as I've said before this isn't an exact science – if you're just starting out with the whole juicing thing, you may want to tip the balance a little more in favour of something sweeter, maybe 45% Beauty and 50% Base. However, this is just until your taste buds get with the programme as high-sugar juices, even though completely natural, can still play havoc with your blood sugar levels!

Feed the smaller, brawnier items through first along with the softer fruits and veggies as they need something firmer to flush them through the juicer.

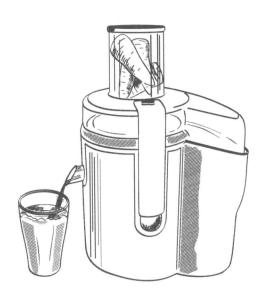

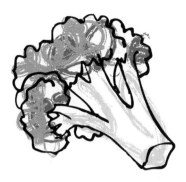

Remember to chew your juice – swoosh it around your mouth, blending it with that enzyme-rich saliva to help keep digestion in tip-top shape.

1 – DETOX DELIGHT SHOT

Spinach / a big handful
Apple / 2 crunchy variety
Mint / small bunch

2 – KILLER CLEANSE

Romaine / 3 heads
Pineapple / 1 cup
Coconut oil / 1 tbsp
(blend with a little hot water to create a milky liquid)

3 – LIVER ELIXIR

Courgette / 3 medium
Pear / 2 crunchy variety
Ginger / ½ inch
chunk or to taste

4 – LEMON ESSENCE

Celery / 5 medium sticks
Beets / 1 medium
Lemon / ½

5 – FULL IMMUNITY

Cucumber / 2 medium
Carrot / 2 medium
Fennel / ½ medium bulb

6 – FAT FLUSH

Kale / big bunch
Melon / 3 cups
Cayenne / to taste

7 – FAST FRIEND

Broccoli / 3 cups
Watermelon /
3 cups – with skin
Coriander / small bunch

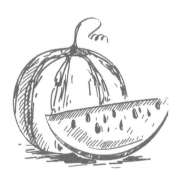

MOTIVATIONAL VIDEOS

We all need a little boost every so often and watching motivational videos online is an inspirational way to feel uplifted and light. They can encourage us to take action, become more aware of our emotions and help us learn and grow. Here are a few of my favourites on YouTube.

Jill Bolte Taylor – TED talk

Live simply so others can simply live

Lizzie Velasquez – TED talk

Caroline Casey – TED Talk

Lillie Mac Cloud First Audition

Stand By Me – Playing For Change

Escaping Earth with Morgan Freeman

About Time – Movie Trailer

The T-Mobile Welcome Back

[Singing Nun] Italian Nun The Voice Italy

ABOUT ANGIE NEWSON

Angie Newson has been at the top of London's health, wellbeing and fitness industry for over two decades. She is a freelance writer, contributing to many UK women's magazines and national newspapers on fitness trends, workouts and anti-ageing secrets. Her first book was *'Get Fit for Free with Yoga and Pilates'*, published by Reader's Digest.

She discovered detoxing whilst in Thailand ten years ago and as well as returning for an annual cleanse, she follows the Daily Detox lifestyle – using all the detox secrets revealed in this book.

She is passionate about healthy eating, Pilates and yoga. She is a fully-qualified Pilates teacher and holds regular classes in London to students of all ages – her eldest client being a lovely lady of 86 full of vitality! She is also teaches yoga and often travels to India and across the globe to deepen her practice and run retreats. She is a teacher-trainer and an assessor for Exercise to Music.

Angie has extensive experience in health club management, formerly General Manager of an award-winning spa in London popular with celebs, media-folk and professionals. She consults on holistic aspects and mind-body studios for top health facilities and is as happy participating in a class as when she's teaching her own session. Angie is constantly learning daily from her peers and her own students!

She has appeared on TV as fitness presenter and expert in various health series and is a Brand Ambassador for fashion-forward, activewear retailer – Sweaty Betty. She enjoys working out every day, has bundles of energy, and loves green tea.

AND THANKS TO ...

My heartfelt thanks goes to ...

DJ for your never-ending wisdom and help writing this book; 'Betty Button' for the laughs and patience; Ruth Patrick for your proofreading skills; my family and dearly-valued friends (you know who you are!) and my beautiful and amazing children, Carly and Theo. And not forgetting my daily reminder to practice love, acceptance and forgiveness – Louie – the best pooch, whose down/up dog poses are simply perfect!

CONNECT WITH ANGIE

TWITTER: @AngieNewson
WEB: AgeproofLiving.com
FACEBOOK: AgeproofLiving

ONE LAST THING ...

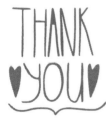

... for purchasing The Detox Factor. I sincerely hope you have enjoyed the home cleansing tips in the book. If you would like to comment or leave a review on Amazon, I'd really appreciate your feedback.

INDEX

A

acid/alkaline balance 16, 55, 73, 75,
    80, 81, 82, 84, 86, 93, 107,
    110, 111, 112, 113, 124
acid reflux 57, 70, 141
AcuMat 75, 117, 139
acupressure 131
acupuncture 117
ACV 18, 46, 51, 54, 80, 97, 130
addiction 41, 69, 84, 92
air purification 138
alcohol 19, 22, 25, 41, 69
    76, 87, 102, 141, 142
alkaline *See* acid/alkaline balance
allergies 23, 56, 86, 102, 104
aluminium 120, 130
Alzheimer's Disease 37, 38
    70, 86, 120, 124, 141
amalgam fillings 23, 38
amino acids 51, 141
anaemia 73, 141
anti-ageing 7, 20, 26, 48, 58, 64, 71, 72
    84, 88, 112, 125, 136, 137, 149
antibacterial 73, 104, 125
antibiotics 18, 23, 41, 55, 113
antidepressant 31
anti-inflammatory 58, 78, 121, 123
antioxidant 38, 39, 51, 58, 61, 65, 71
    74, 77, 88, 92 119, 121, 123,124
apple cider vinegar *See* ACV
aromatherapy 101, 131, 138
arthritis 58, 87, 141
Ashtanga yoga 133, 134
asthma 23, 93, 96, 102, 104, 106, 124
avocado 43, 95, 135
Ayurveda 39, 58, 59, 60, 131, 141

B

beets 73, 119, 147
bentonite clay 86
bicarbonate of soda 97
Bikram yoga 7, 133
blueberries 38, 124

bone broth 50, 59
breathing 15, 64, 70, 92, 93, 95, 100,
    101, 106, 107, 115, 116, 126, 129, 134
Buddhism 33
Buteyko Method 100
cacao 38, 65
caffeine 19, 35, 69, 87, 123
calcium 51, 81, 86, 117, 123
cancer 36, 38, 56, 61, 81, 86, 92, 119, 128, 130
candida 23, 125, 141
cardiovascular disease 38, 66, 71, 77, 94
castor oil pack 88, 89
cayenne pepper 58, 61, 72, 78, 118, 145, 147
celery 37, 52, 119, 145, 147
cellulite 23, 51
chakras 33, 39, 141
chanting 33, 70, 71, 124, 128
chilli *See* cayenne pepper
chocolate 22, 58
cholesterol 41, 42, 77, 80, 88, 119, 122
circulation 40, 58, 64, 92, 95
    115, 121, 136, 137, 139
cirrhosis 76, 87, 141
clutter 16, 45, 46, 137
coconut oil 43, 61, 63, 65, 118, 132, 135, 147
coffee 22, 87, 92, 123, 124
colds 5, 23, 41, 73, 95, 99, 103, 104, 137
collagen 51, 128
colon 14, 19, 49, 50, 56, 59, 61, 63, 71, 87, 142
constipation 19, 23, 49, 50
    52, 61, 69, 77, 87, 142
cortisol 26, 29, 48, 142
cranberries 38, 76, 119, 124, 125, 145
cucumber 57, 112, 119, 120, 145, 147
cupping 103

D

dairy 22, 72, 110, 118, 123, 126, 130
dandelion 81, 86, 87, 119, 145
daylight 15, 31, 35
declutter 45
dementia 37, 86
deodorants 17, 129, 130
depression 23, 27, 28, 31, 32, 42, 56, 124, 139

NOTES

9139569R10086

Printed in Great Britain
by Amazon.co.uk, Ltd.,
Marston Gate.